Atlas of Pediatric CTA of Coronary Artery Anomalies

Randy Ray Richardson

Atlas of Pediatric CTA of Coronary Artery Anomalies

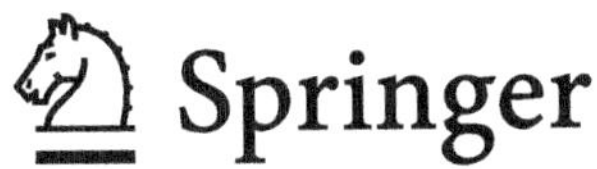

Springer

Randy Ray Richardson, MD
Creighton University School of Medicine
St. Joseph's Hospital and Medical Center
Phoenix, AZ, USA

ISBN 978-3-030-28086-4   ISBN 978-3-030-28087-1   (eBook)
https://doi.org/10.1007/978-3-030-28087-1

This Springer imprint is published by the registered company Springer Nature Switzerland AG
The registered company address is: Gewerbestrasse 11, 6330 Cham, Switzerland

I would like to dedicate this book to the memory of Dr. Janet Strife, MD. In my opinion, one of the great leaders in radiology passed away on May 8, 2019. If anyone ever asked me what kind of radiologist I would like to be, I would always have answered that I want to be like Janet Strife. Janet was Chief of Radiology while I was a fellow at Children's Hospital in Cincinnati. She was President of the Society for Pediatric Radiology in 2000 and President of the Program Directors in Radiology in 2003–2004. She had many peer-reviewed publications, textbooks, and chapters on pediatric radiology.

I am sure her great knowledge base and leadership experience helped to make her a great mentor, but I don't remember reading any of her journal articles or books or even any of the lectures she gave.

What I remember is how she sparked my interest in cardiac imaging by allowing me to sit with her and read the cardiac catheterizations for babies and children with congenital heart disease.

What I remember was her invitation to thanksgiving dinner and other holidays at her home with all of the other radiology fellows where we sat and enjoyed the company of Janet, Fred, and her family.

What I remember is her comforting my teary-eyed wife who was frustrated when we moved to Cincinnati because we couldn't find a place to live.

I think the word "mentor" is often overused and underperformed. I never remember Dr. Strife using the word "mentor" to describe herself, but she was one of the greatest mentors I have ever known.

Her legacy will live on in the lives of many, like me, who have benefitted from her leadership, teaching, and mentorship.

Preface

The *Atlas of Pediatric CTA of Coronary Artery Anomalies* is a concise visual guide to the imaging of coronary artery anomalies in infants and children. Imaging plays an ever-increasing role in diagnosis, preoperative planning, and postoperative management for children with congenital and acquired heart disease. Coronary artery anomalies, when present, need to be imaged and understood before surgical intervention to avoid potential morbidity and mortality. The book, therefore, focuses on the utilization of advanced CT imaging for pediatric patients with coronary arteries artery anomalies which are distinct from adult patients, with an emphasis on techniques for lowering radiation, protocols for imaging infants and children, and recommendations for most appropriate studies that should decrease the time and cost of imaging these patients.

Coronary artery anomalies are well described in the adult literature. What makes this book unique is that it sees the relation of the coronary artery anomalies to common and uncommon congenital heart defects. The other unique feature of this atlas is the visualization of these anomalies in infants where the coronary arteries are often 1–2 mm in diameter. We feel fortunate to have accumulated one of the largest collections of coronary artery anomalies for infants and children.

Our hope is that this information may be used to teach physicians in training who are interested in the fields of pediatrics, cardiology, and radiology and as a review for physicians studying for maintenance of certification and board examinations. We also feel that this book will stimulate new ideas for imaging in infants and children by the many physicians who will continue to improve and evolve the quality and safe treatment of this subset of patients.

I want to give credit to the wide variety of physicians who have contributed to this publication through regular conferences, discussions, lectures, and research collaboration:

- Ernerio Albollras, MD
- Shabib Alhadheri, MD
- Deepti Bhat, MD
- Kevin Brady, MD
- Deepa Prasad, MD
- Rahel Zubairi, MD
- Randall Fortuna, MD
- David Frakes, PhD
- Pankaj Jain, MD
- Olga Kalinkin, MD
- Lawrence (Larney) Lilien, MD
- Dan Miga, MD
- Hursh Naik, MD
- John Nigro, MD
- Jonathan Plascencia, PhD
- Stephen Pophal, MD

- Mitchell Ross, MD
- Justin Ryan, PhD
- Janet Strife, MD
- Eunice Yoon, MD

Phoenix, AZ, USA

Randy Ray Richardson, MD

Contents

Contributors

Elizabeth C. England, MSIV Creighton University School of Medicine Phoenix Regional Campus, Phoenix, AZ, USA

Dylan J. Hoyt, MSIV Creighton University School of Medicine Phoenix Regional Campus, Phoenix, AZ, USA

Olga Kalinkin, MD Creighton University School of Medicine Phoenix Regional Campus, St. Joseph's Hospital and Medical Center, Phoenix, AZ, USA

Randy Ray Richardson, MD Creighton University School of Medicine, St. Joseph's Hospital and Medical Center, Phoenix, AZ, USA

Recent advances in multidetector CT (MDCT) technology have revolutionized cardiovascular imaging in children with complex congenital heart disease. Fast scanning times and high-quality evaluation of both complex cardiac and coronary anatomy have enabled computed tomography angiography (CTA) to aid in patient management and treatment planning. For infants with congenital heart disease, an electrocardiogram or ECG-gated cardiac CTA is the modality of choice for imaging the coronary arteries, cardiac morphology, the airway, and extracardiac vascular structures, supplemented by functional analysis of left ventricular ejection fraction and cardiac wall motion. To fully utilize the advantages of cardiac CTA, it is important to consider radiation exposure and to optimize scanning techniques. Currently, there are two accepted cardiac CTA scanning techniques for infants and small children with congenital heart disease: retrospective and prospective ECG-gated scanning.

1.1 MDCT Technique

All cardiac CTA examinations are performed with the MDCT scanners. General anesthesia is administered routinely in infants less than 1 year of age to optimize the scans. After being intubated by the anesthesiologist, the patient is transferred to the CT scanner with an intravenous line and ECG leads in place. During CTA examination, precise communication and coordination between the radiologist, the anesthesiologist, the CT technologist, and the nurse are needed to produce the optimal scan. The radiologist's discussion with the cardiologist is important to optimize the protocol; however, the standard MDCT protocol allows covering the cardiac, coronary, and extra-cardiac pathology in infants and young children. Beta-blockers typically are not used to decrease the heart rate in children with congenital heart disease. Nitrates are also not applied in infants and young children. When possible, an intravenous line is positioned in the left arm in order to identify the left superior vena cava.

Iodinated contrast medium is used at 1 mL/lb of body weight, with an injection rate of 0.7 mL/sec independently of the type of retrospective or prospective ECG-gating technique. After obtaining the scout via the chest, the technologist identifies the appropriated scan coverage. While the anesthesiologist assists with holding the breathing, the technologist begins the scan when contrast material has filled the left ventricle. The patient is scanned in a craniocaudal direction starting at the level of the subclavian artery and ending at the level of the diaphragm.

An ECG-gated CTA scan is acquired with prospective or retrospective protocol. With a GE 64-slice MDCT detector size of 0.625 mm, a single rotation of scanner gantry provides 40 mm of coverage. The length of the entire chest to be covered is typically 100 mm. Temporal resolution is affected by gantry speed rotation and pitch. The gantry speed is set at a 0.35-second rotation and defined by scanner mechanical factors. For infants and small children, the tube voltage value is used at 80 peak kilovoltage (kVp). Adjusted according to body weight, the tube current varies from institution to institution and may range from 10 to 40 mA/kg [1, 2].

1.2 Retrospective Scanning

Retrospective scanning provides not only anatomic morphologic data but also functional information about left ventricular ejection fraction. During ECG-gated retrospective scanning, the x-ray beam is turned on for the entire R R interval of the cardiac cycle while spiral scanning continues during table motion to cover the anatomy (Fig. 1.1). ECG retrospective gating in adults uses a low pitch value of 0.2. Low pitch is a requirement in cardiac imaging to collect sufficient data of attenuation measurements at all spatial locations in the heart and to scan during all phases of the cardiac cycle. The pitch in retrospective scanning depends on the heart rate. Pitch normally falls in the range of 0.2 to 0.24 for infants with heart rates above 100 bpm. The current in retrospective scanning is set at 250 to 300 mA.

© Springer Nature Switzerland AG 2020
R. R. Richardson, *Atlas of Pediatric CTA of Coronary Artery Anomalies*, https://doi.org/10.1007/978-3-030-28087-1_1

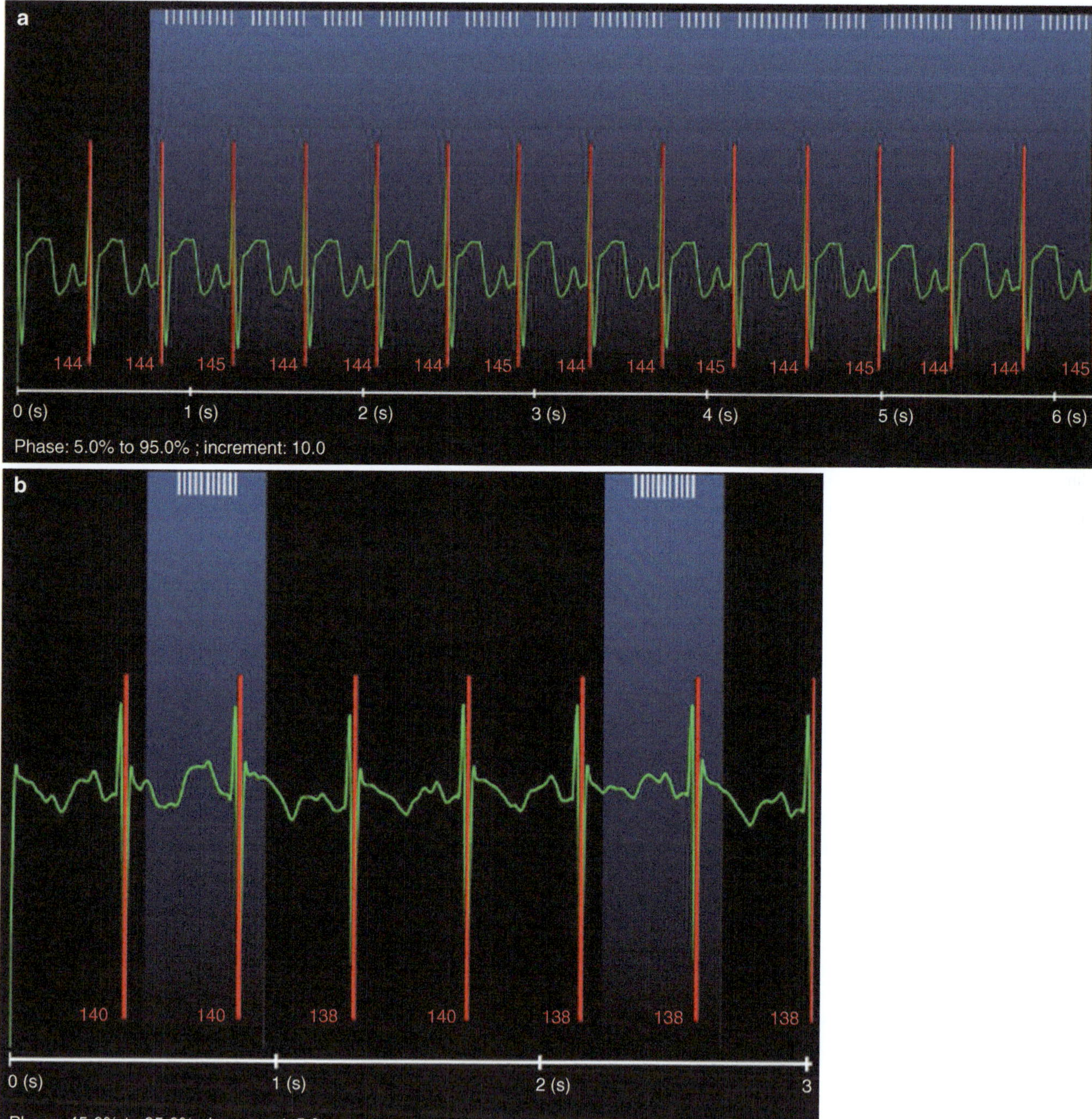

Fig. 1.1 (**a**) Retrospective ECG-gated cardiac CTA scan diagram. The x-ray beam (*blue*) is on throughout the entire cardiac cycle during helical scanning. (**b**) Prospective ECG-gated cardiac CTA scan diagram. The x-ray beam (*blue*) is on only during the end diastolic phase of the cardiac cycle during helical scanning

1.3   Prospective Scanning

The vast majority of scanning can and should be done using the prospective ECG-triggered scanning technique, even in small children and infants with very fast heart rates. This technique uses a non-spiral "step-and-shoot" axial scanning process in which the x-ray beam is on for a short period of time and is turned off as the table moves. This cycle step-and-shoot repeats several times to cover the entire cardiac anatomy. Typically, end diastole is the time of a relatively motionless heart window for the coronary arteries in adults, with optimal visualization of coronary arteries between 70%

and 80% of the of phases of the cardiac cycle. In infants, the optimal time of decreased motion of coronary arteries typically is during the end systole, at 45% to 55% of the cardiac cycle. Relatively high infants' heart rates are translated into the small R-R interval. Therefore additional sampling of cardiac cycle data is achieved by application of padding to the short acquisition time captured up to 50% of the cardiac cycle data to evaluate the coronary arteries (Fig. 1.2). The padding turns the x-ray tube on 175 msec before the required acquisition time and leaves it on for an additional 175 msec, allowing more imaged data from the cardiac cycle to be obtained (Fig. 1.3). This supplementary data is useful for calculation of the left ventricular ejection fraction and functional analysis of the left ventricle. The tube current is adjusted according the

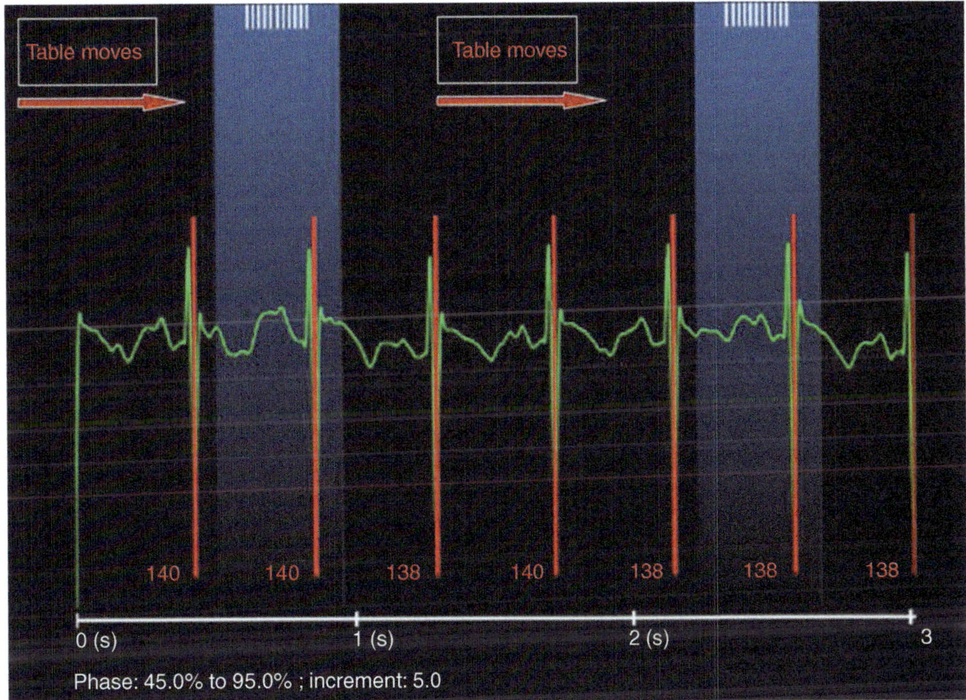

Fig. 1.2 Prospective ECG-gated cardiac CTA scan technique diagram. The x-ray beam (*blue*) is on during the end systolic (45%) to diastolic (95%) phases of the R-R interval. This rapid heart rate of 140 bpm allows acquisition of a greater than 50% portion of the cardiac cycle data so that functional information can be obtained with post-processing

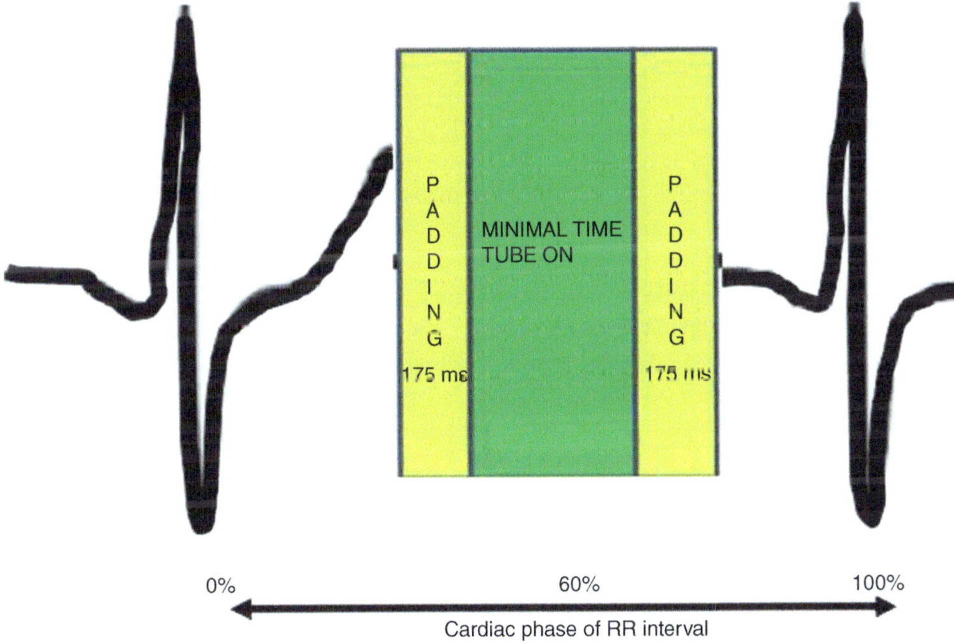

Fig. 1.3 Scheme of padding. Scan time during diastole is equal to the minimal time tube on (*green*) plus padding of 175 msec (*yellow*) used before and after to acquire more data by adding more cardiac phases

Table 1.1 Radiograph tube current is adjusted according to the body weight adjustments in prospectively gated cardiac CTA scanning

Infant body weight, *lb*	Current, *mA*
4–13	240
13–16	400
16–25	460

Table 1.2 Comparison of retrospective versus prospective ECG-gated cardiac CTA scanning techniques

Retrospective ECG-gated scan	Prospective ECG-gated scan
Scans the entire R-R interval	Scans a variable portion of the R-R interval (end systolic-early diastolic phases) with added padding time
X-ray beam is *on* the entire scanning time	X-ray beam is *not* on the entire scanning time
No padding	Padding may be used to increased sampling during the cardiac cycle to obtain functional information
Higher radiation dose	Lower radiation dose

patient's body weight, with three protocol settings of 240, 400, and 460 mA (Table 1.1).

Table 1.2 shows the differences between prospective and retrospective scanning.

1.4 Radiation Dose

Children are more sensitive than adults to the effects of ionizing radiation; therefore, it is essential to balance image quality with radiation dose delivered when performing CTA in children. It is imperative to apply the ALARA (As Low As Reasonably Achievable) principle for infants and small children by using appropriate low kilovolt peak and low adjusted milliamperes to the patient's weight. Published studies comparing retrospective with prospective ECG-gated scanning techniques have reported radiation dose savings ranging from two to four times with prospective ECG-gated techniques [1–4]. Less than 1 MSV (millisievert) radiation doses were achieved with the prospective ECG-gated protocols. On the contrary, retrospective ECG-gated scanning yields higher radiation doses, estimated to be around 3 to 10 MSV, even with the low-dose technique [5–10].

Adaptive statistical iterative reconstruction, a unique CT reconstruction algorithm with matrix algebra used to selectively identify and subtract noise from the image, is another technical tool that may be used to lower the radiation dose for children. The result is less noise or the same amount of noise with less radiation exposure [8–11].

1.5 Cardiac CTA Data Post-processing and Analysis

At our institution, all acquired image data are reconstructed into the section thickness of 0.625 mm and a section interval of 0.625 mm with use of a small cardiac field of view. The lung window is reconstructed at a 2.5-mm section. All obtained axial images are transferred to an external workstation, where they are reconstructed with multiplanar reformation, volume rendering, and maximum intensity projections. The protocol parameters used at our institution are described in detail in Table 1.3.

Table 1.3 Summary of retrospective and prospective ECG-gated MDCT cardiac CTA protocols in infants for a 64-slice GE scanner

Parameter	Retrospective ECG-gated scan	Prospective ECG-gated scan
Contrast	Iodinated contrast medium (iopamidol, 300 mg/mL) is used at 1 mL/lb of body weight with an injection speed of 0.7 mL/sec	Iodinated contrast medium (iopamidol, 300 mg/mL) is used at 1 mL/lb of body weight with an injection speed of 0.7 mL/sec
Peak kilovoltage	80 kVp	80 kVp
Current	Set at 300 mA	Selected by weight at 240, 400, or 460 mA
Scan time during R-R interval	Entire interval	50–75% phases of R-R interval + padding
Pitch	0.2–0.24	None
Padding	None	175 msec
Rotation, *sec*	0.35	0.35
Collimation versus reconstruction interval/*mm*	0.6	0.6
Slice thickness, *mm*	0.625	0.625
Field of view	100 mm	100 mm

References

1. Jin KN, Park EA, Shin CI, Lee W, Chung JW, Park JH. Retrospective versus prospective ECG-gated dual-source CT in pediatric patients with congenital heart diseases: comparison of image quality and radiation dose. Int J Cardiovasc Imaging. 2010;26(Suppl 1):63–73.
2. Hollingsworth CL, Yoshizumi TT, Frush DP, Chan FP, Toncheva G, Nguyen G, et al. Pediatric cardiac-gated CT angiography: assessment of radiation dose. Am J Roentgenol. 2007;189:12–8.
3. Paul JF, Rohnean A, Elfassy E, Sigal-Cinqualbre A. Radiation dose for thoracic and coronary step-and-shoot CT using a 128-slice dual-source machine in infants and small children with congenital heart disease. Pediatr Radiol. 2011;41:244–9.
4. Paul JF, Rohnean A, Sigal-Cinqualbre A. Multidetector CT for congenital heart patients: what a paediatric radiologist should know. Pediatr Radiol. 2010;40:869–75.
5. Hirai N, Horiguchi J, Fujioka C, Kiguchi M, Yamamoto H, Matsuura N, et al. Prospective versus retrospective ECG-gated 64 detector coronary CT angiography: assessment of image quality, stenosis, and radiation dose. Radiology. 2008;248:424–30.
6. Kuettner A, Gehann B, Spolnik J, Koch A, Achenbach S, Weyand M, et al. Strategies for dose-optimized imaging in pediatric cardiac dual source CT. Rofo. 2009;181:339–48.
7. Huang B, Law MW, Mak HK, Kwok SP, Khong PL. Pediatric 64-MDCT coronary angiography with ECG-modulated tube current: radiation dose and cancer risk. Am J Roentgenol. 2009;193:539–44.
8. Al-Mousily F, Shifrin RY, Fricker FJ, Feranec N, Quinn NS, Chandran A. Use of 320-detector computed tomographic angiography for infants and young children with congenital heart disease. Pediatr Cardiol. 2011;32:426–32.
9. Pages J, Buls N, Osteaux M. CT doses in children: a multicentre study. Br J Radiol. 2003;76(911):803–11.
10. Deak PD, Smal Y, Kalender WA. Multisection CT protocols: sex- and age-specific conversion factors used to determine effective dose from dose-length product. Radiology. 2010;257:158–66.
11. Li X, Samei E, Segars WP, Sturgeon GM, Colsher JG, Frush DP. Patient-specific radiation dose and cancer risk for pediatric chest CT. Radiology. 2011;259:862–74.

Many normal variants of the coronary arteries exist. In this chapter we will only review coronary artery dominance and a few other common coronary artery normal variants. Other normal variants are described throughout the other chapters of the book.

2.1 Coronary Dominance

Coronary artery dominance is determined by the artery that supplies the posterior descending artery (PDA) and the posterolateral branch (PLB). The PDA courses in the posterior interventricular groove and supplies the inferior interven-tricular septum. The PLB courses laterally, also supplying the inferior myocardium. There are three classic possibilities for coronary dominance: (1) right dominance (70%), in which the PDA and PLB arise from the right coronary circu-lation, (2) left dominance (10%), in which the PDA and PLB arise from the left coronary circulation (more typically the circumflex artery [CX]), or (3) codominance (20%), in which the PDA and PLB arise variably from both the right and left coronary circulations. A variety of possibilities exist with a codominant circulation. The inferior wall may be supplied by a number of small branches from the left anterior descend-ing artery (LAD), the CX artery, and the right coronary artery (RCA)(Figs. 2.1, 2.2, 2.3, and 2.4).

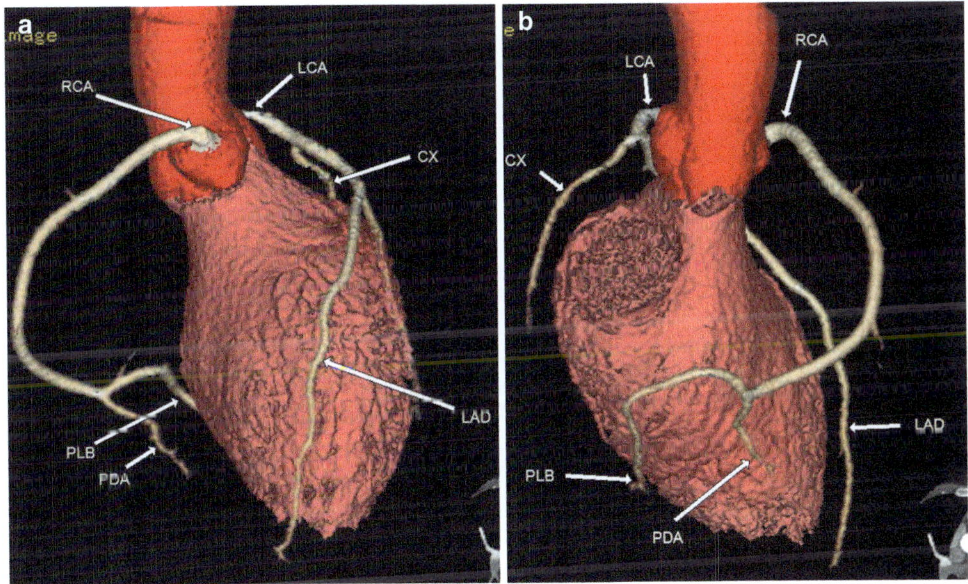

Fig. 2.1 Frontal (**a**) and posterior (**b**) views from color-coded 3D volume-rendered images from a cardiac computed tomography angiography (CTA) shows a classic right dominant coronary artery system with both the PDA and the PLB arising from the distal right coronary artery (RCA). Left circulation coronary arteries are also labeled (LCA, LAD, and CX)

© Springer Nature Switzerland AG 2020

R. R. Richardson, *Atlas of Pediatric CTA of Coronary Artery Anomalies*, https://doi.org/10.1007/978-3-030-28087-1_2

Fig. 2.2 Frontal (**a**) and posterior (**b**) views from color-coded 3D volume-rendered image from a cardiac CTA shows a left dominant coronary artery system with both the PDA and the PLB arising from the distal circumflex coronary artery (CX). Other coronary arteries are also labeled (LCA, LAD, and RCA)

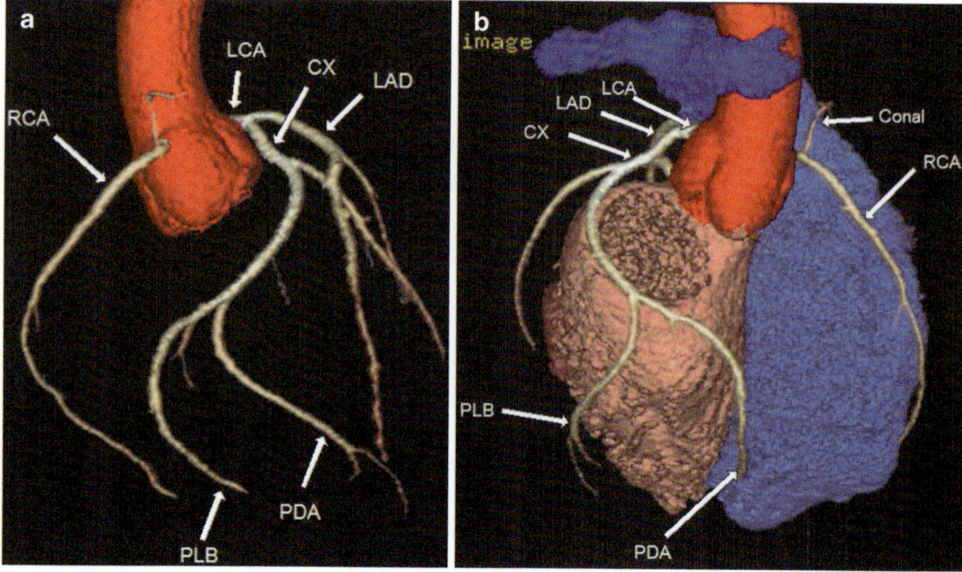

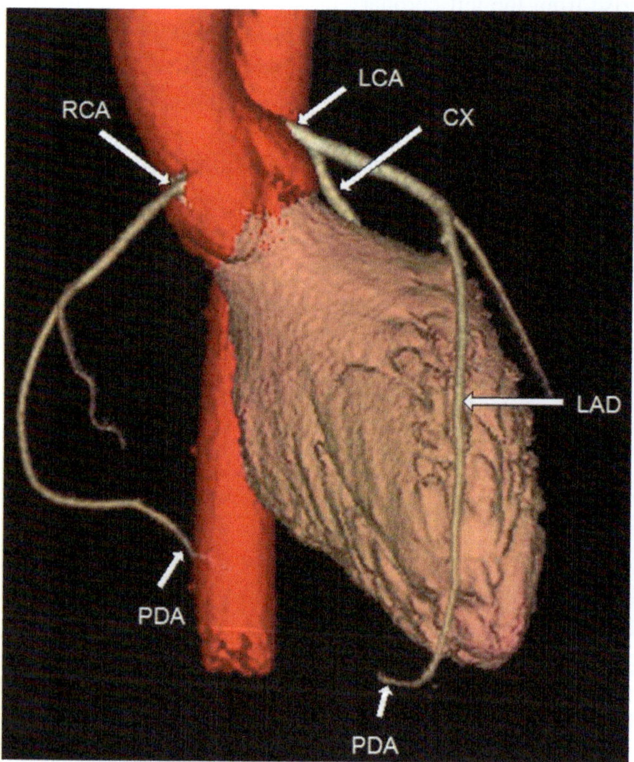

Fig. 2.3 A frontal view from a color-coded 3D volume-rendered image from a cardiac CTA shows a codominant coronary artery system with the PDA arising from the right coronary artery (RCA) and the PLB arising from the left anterior descending coronary artery (LAD). Other coronary arteries are also labeled (LCA and CX)

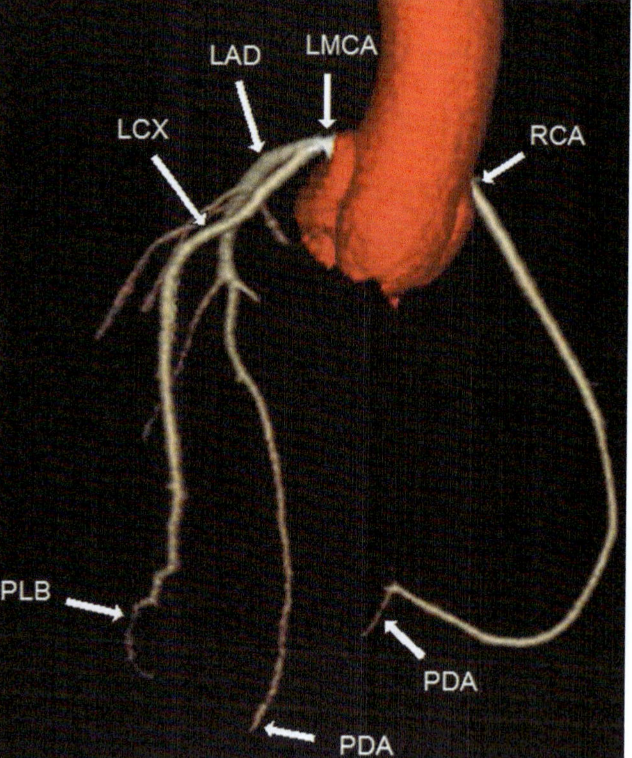

Fig. 2.4 A posterior view from a color-coded 3D volume-rendered image from a cardiac CTA shows a codominant coronary artery system with the PDA arising from the right coronary artery (RCA) and the PLB arising from the circumflex coronary artery (CX). Also, notice that the left anterior descending coronary artery (LAD) supplies a portion of the inferior wall with a duplicated PDA arising distally. The left coronary artery (LCA) is also labeled

2.2   Ramus Intermedius

In this normal variant there is a trifurcation of the left coronary artery into the LAD, CX, and a ramus intermedius. The ramus intermedius typically acts as a diagonal or marginal branch and supplies the inferolateral wall of the left ventricle (Fig. 2.5).

2.3   Myocardial Bridging

Typically, coronary arteries are surrounded by fat in the epicardial space around the heart. Myocardial bridging is seen when the coronary artery deviates from its normal course and dips into the myocardium of the heart. Compression of the coronary artery with myocardial bridging is certainly a risk, but the vast majority of the time when the coronary artery courses into the myocardium, there is no significant narrowing, and the patient is asymptomatic [5]. Myocardial bridging has been found in up to 25% of patients by computed tomography (CT). The majority of cases of normal variant myocardial bridging involve the middle LAD (Fig. 2.6).

2.4   Shepherd Crook Deformity

A shepherd crook deformity is a normal variant in which the proximal RCA takes a superior course and then loops back down into its normal position in the right atrioventricular groove (Fig. 2.7).

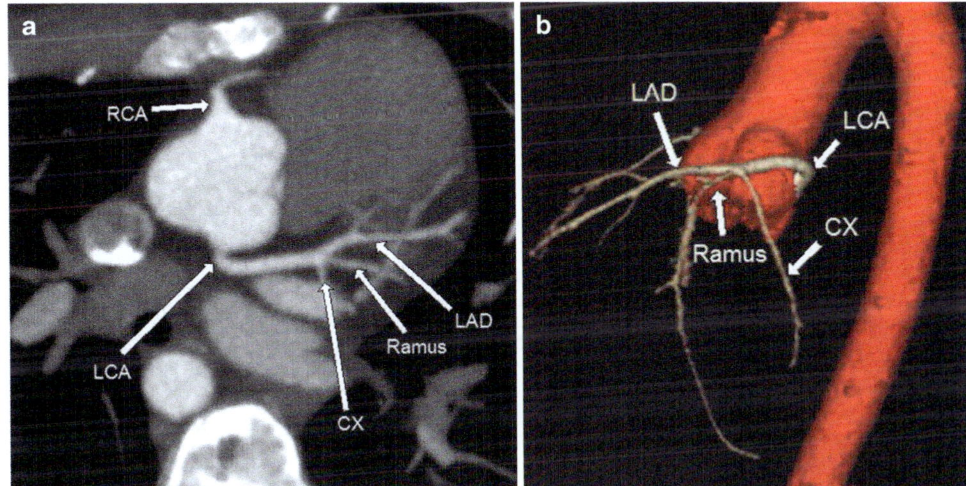

Fig. 2.5 Axial oblique maximum intensity projection (MIP) (**a**) and color-coded 3D volume-rendered images (**b**) from a cardiac CTA showing trifurcation of the left coronary artery (LCA). The left anterior descending (LAD) and circumflex arteries (CX) arise normally, but a third vessel is seen arising centrally that is consistent with a normal variant ramus intermedius (ramus)

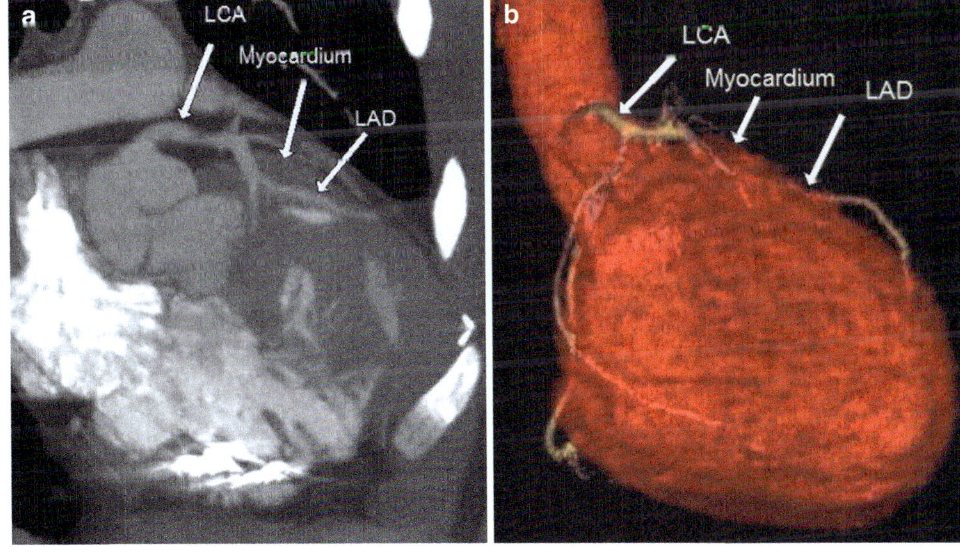

Fig. 2.6 Coronal oblique MIP (**a**) and color-coded 3D volume-rendered images (**b**) from a cardiac CTA show the course of the left anterior descending artery (LAD) through the myocardium of the left ventricle, which is consistent with myocardial bridging. No significant coronary narrowing was seen even during systole, and the patient was asymptomatic

Fig. 2.7 Color-coded 3D volume-rendered image from a cardiac CTA in an infant (*left*) with a digital artistic rendering of the ascending aorta and the right coronary artery (RCA; *right*) shows a normal variant looped course of the proximal RCA on both volume-rendered image and artistic rendering, consistent with a shepherd crook normal variant

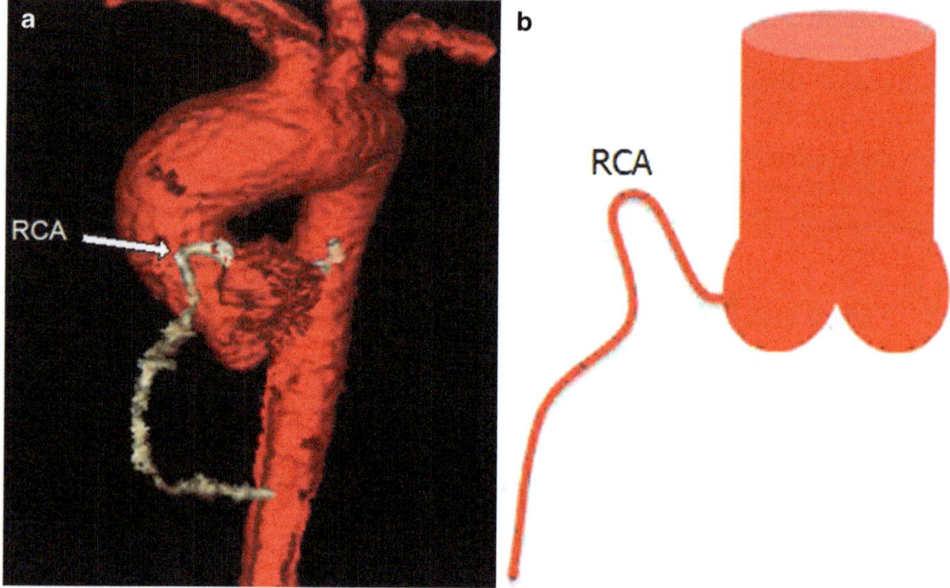

References

1. Shriki JE, Shinbane JS, Rashid MA, Hindoyan A, Withey JG, DeFrance A, et al. Identifying, characterizing, and classifying congenital anomalies of the coronary arteries. Radiographics. 2012;32:453–68.
2. Yu M, Zhang Y, Li Y, Li M, Li W, Zhang J. Assessment of myocardial bridge by cardiac CT: intracoronary transluminal attenuation gradient derived from diastolic phase predicts systolic compression. Korean J Radiol. 2017;18:655–63.
3. Young PM, Gerber TC, Williamson EE, Julsrud PR, Herfkens RJ. Cardiac imaging: part 2, normal, variant, and anomalous configurations of the coronary vasculature. Am J Roentgenol. 2011;197:816–26.
4. Angelini P. Normal and anomalous coronary arteries: definitions and classification. Am Heart J. 1989;117:418–34.
5. Angelini P. Coronary artery anomalies–current clinical issues: definitions, classification, incidence, clinical relevance, and treatment guidelines. Tex Heart Inst J. 2002;29:271–8.

Normally the right and left coronary arteries arise from the corresponding right and left coronary sinuses, respectively. Coronary arteries typically arise from the coronary sinuses closest to the pulmonary artery. Embryologically, the coronary arteries develop in the epicardial atrioventricular and interventricular grooves and then connect to the aorta late in their development. There is a wide spectrum of where along the coronary artery ostium their origin can occur on the path of the coronary sinus. The coronary ostium may normally arise up to 5 mm above the aortic sinotubular junction. There is also a wide range in the number of coronary arteries that may arise. Origins include a single coronary artery, two origins from the same sinus, multiple origins from multiple sinuses, oblique origins frequently seen with an intramural course, and high origins along the sinotubular junction. Right or left coronary arteries may arise from the contralateral coronary artery as well. These anomalies are briefly discussed here and then more fully examined in the chapter on coronary artery course anomalies (*see* Chap. 5). Coronary origins may be normal but have an unusual appearance in infants and children with congenital heart disease. We will review a few of these cases in this chapter.

3.1   Normal Coronary Artery Origin

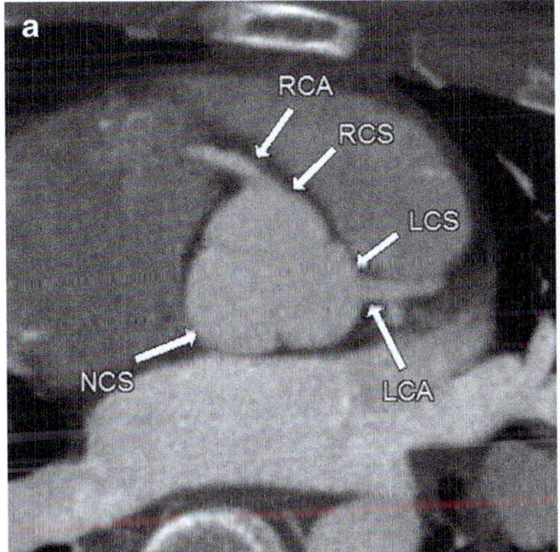

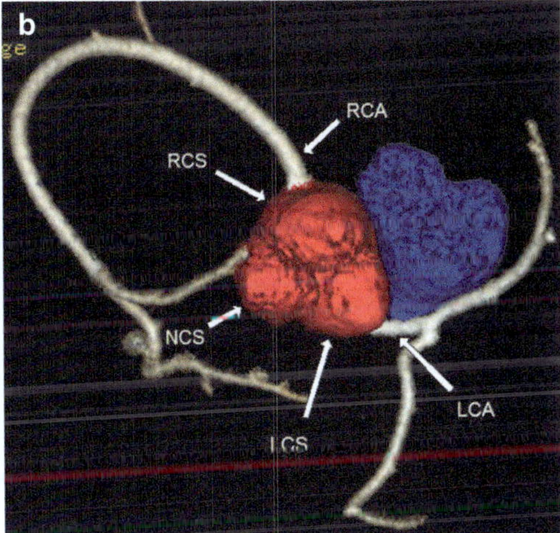

Fig. 3.1 Maximum intensity projection (MIP) (**a**) and 3D color-coded images (**b**) in a patient with normal coronary artery origins of the right (RCA) and left (LCA) coronary arteries from the right and left coronary sinuses and no coronary origin from the non coronary sinus (NCS). Notice the position of the pulmonary artery (*blue*). Coronary arteries typically arise from the coronary sinuses closest to the pulmonary artery

© Springer Nature Switzerland AG 2020

R. R. Richardson, *Atlas of Pediatric CTA of Coronary Artery Anomalies*, https://doi.org/10.1007/978-3-030-28087-1_3

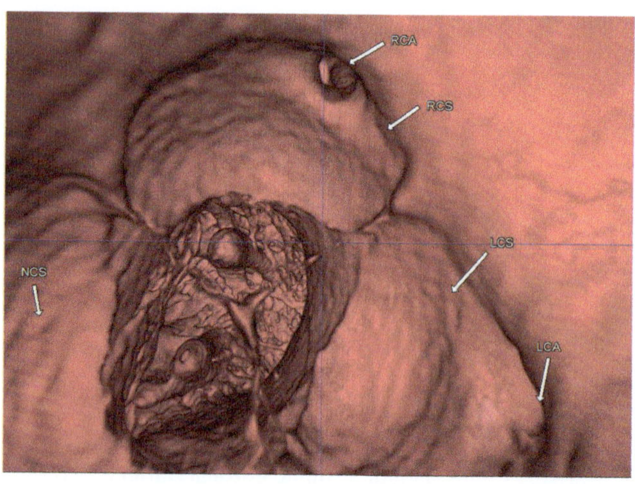

Fig. 3.2 Single image from an intraluminal 3D view from cardiac computed tomography angiography (CTA) shows the typical normal anatomy, with the right coronary artery (RCA) arising from the right coronary sinus (RCS) and the left coronary artery (LCA) arising from the left coronary sinus (LCS); there is no origin from the non-coronary sinus (NCS)

3.2 Single Coronary Artery Origin

Single coronary arteries are rare anomalies and are often associated with other congenital heart defects such as pulmonary atresia, tetralogy of Fallot, and truncus arteriosus. Lipton and colleagues created a classification that describes their origin from the sinus of Valsalva, the course of the vessel, and the transverse trunk. Most patients with a single coronary artery anomaly are asymptomatic. Single coronary arteries that course between the outflow tracts may cause atypical chest pain or syncope with exercise, and the patient may develop an arrhythmia or myocardial infarction. Treatment of single coronary artery anomalies is controversial. Most treatment plans are conservative, using medical management and imaging to assess for potential complications. Surgical treatment has included angioplasty and stenting as well as coronary artery bypass. In this chapter we will show the classic anomalous origins of single coronary arteries from all coronary sinuses and from the sinotubular junction.

3.2.1 Single Coronary Artery Origin from the Right Coronary Sinus

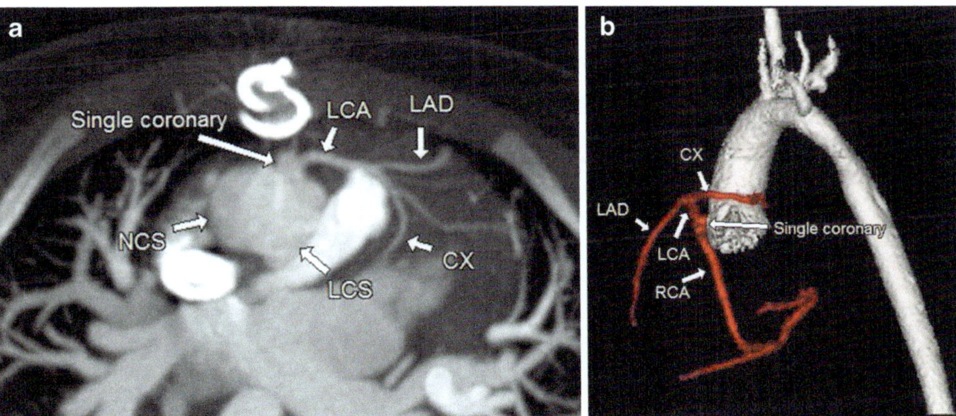

Fig. 3.3 MIP (**a**) and 3D color-coded images (**b**) from a cardiac CTA in an infant status post-repair of the Tetralogy of Fallot. Images show a single coronary artery arising from the right coronary sinus (RCS). Notice that the left coronary artery (LCA) has a prepulmonary course and then divides into the left anterior descending (LAD) and circumflex (CX) arteries. The non-coronary sinus (NCS) and left coronary sinus (LCS) are shown

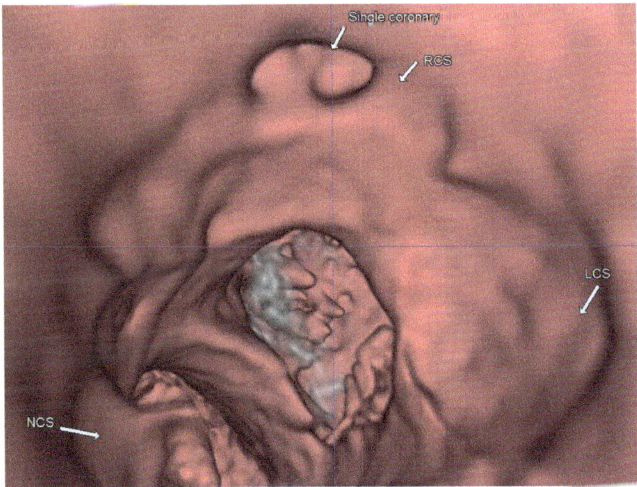

Fig. 3.4 Intraluminal 3D reconstruction from a cardiac CTA in an infant status post-repair of the Tetralogy of Fallot. The single image shows a single coronary artery arising from the right coronary sinus (RCS). The non-coronary sinus (NCS) and left coronary sinus (LCS) are shown with no coronary artery origins

3.2.2 Single Coronary Artery Origin from the Left Coronary Sinus

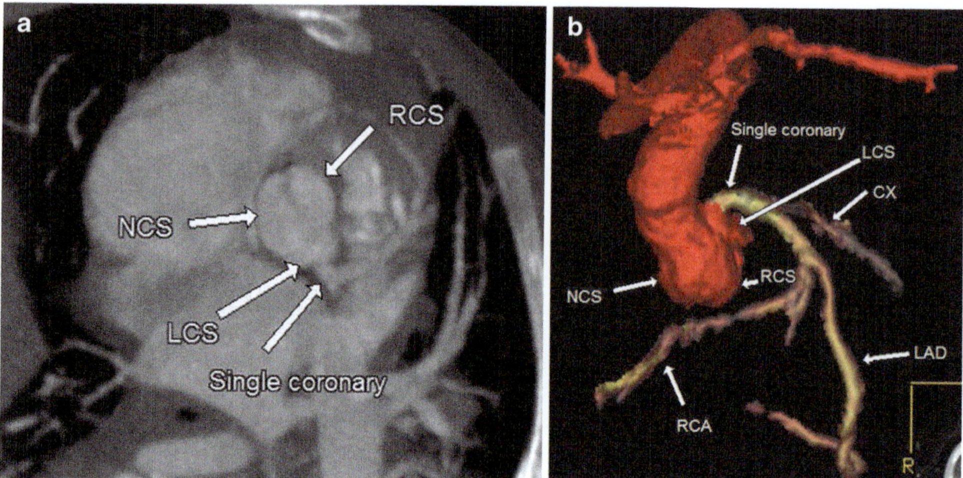

Fig. 3.5 MIP (**a**) and 3D color-coded images (**b**) from a cardiac CTA in an infant with congenital heart disease. Images show a single coronary artery arising from the left coronary sinus (LCS). Notice that the right coronary artery (RCA) arises from the left anterior descending artery (LAD) and has a prepulmonary course. The circumflex (CX) coronary artery is somewhat hypoplastic and arises from the single coronary artery as well. The non-coronary sinus (NCS) and right coronary sinus (RCS) are shown

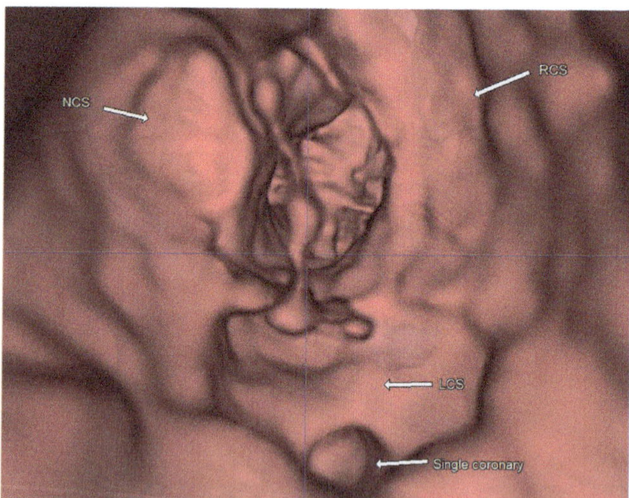

Fig. 3.6 Intraluminal 3D reconstruction from a cardiac CTA in an infant with known congenital heart disease. The single image shows a single coronary artery arising from the right coronary sinus (RCS). The non-coronary sinus (NCS) and right coronary sinus (RCS) are also shown with no coronaries arising from these sinuses

3.2.3 Single Coronary Artery Origin from the Non-coronary Sinus

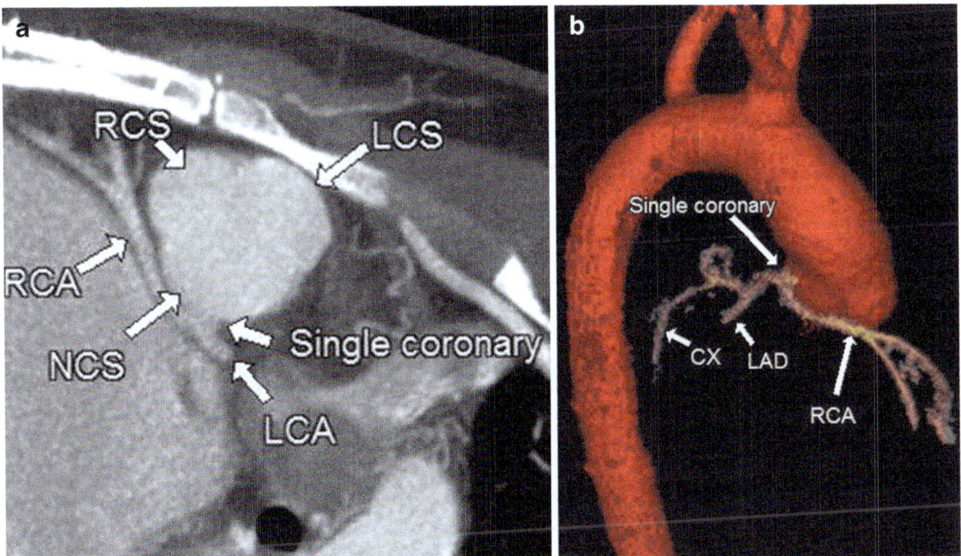

Fig. 3.7 MIP (**a**) and 3D color-coded images (**b**) from a cardiac CTA in an infant with congenital heart disease showing a single coronary artery arising from the non-coronary sinus (NCS). Notice that the left coronary artery (LCA) takes a retro-aortic course before bifurcating into the left anterior descending artery (LAD) and the circumflex (CX) coronary artery. The right coronary artery (RCA) goes directly to the right atrioventricular groove, is somewhat hypoplastic, and arises from the single coronary artery as well. The left coronary sinus (LCS) and right coronary sinus (RCS) are also shown

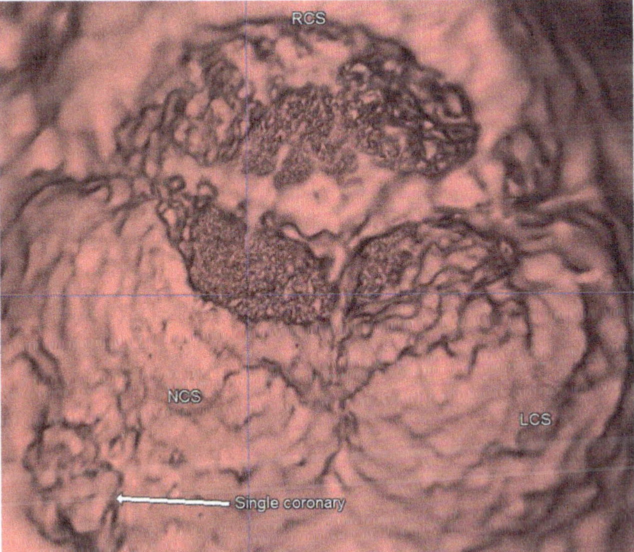

Fig. 3.8 Intraluminal 3D reconstruction from a cardiac CTA in an infant with known congenital heart disease. The single image shows a single coronary artery arising from the non-coronary sinus (NCS). The left and right coronary sinuses (LCS, RCS) are also shown with no coronary artery origins

3.2.4 Single Coronary Artery Origin from the Right Sinotubular Junction

Instead of a single coronary artery origin, the right and left coronary arteries may arise from the same coronary sinus rather than having a single arterial origin as previously discussed. The course of the coronary arteries when this occurs is critical. We will address this course in the following chapter but will show the separate origins from the same sinus here.

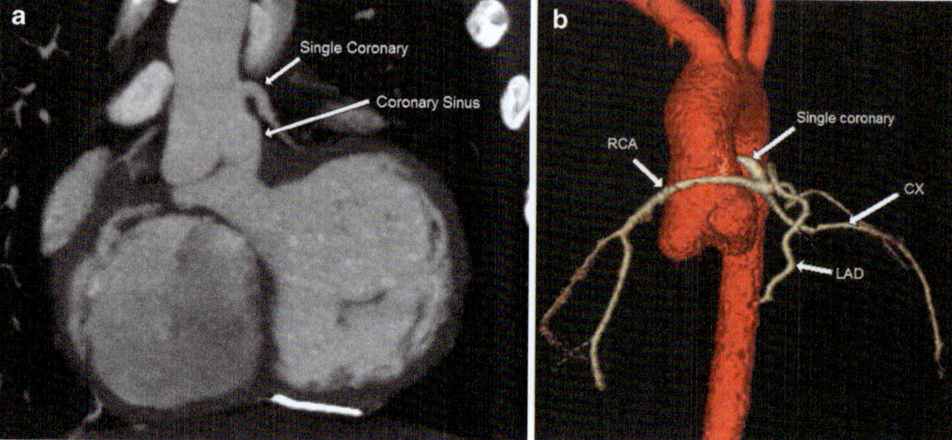

Fig. 3.9 MIP (**a**) and 3D color-coded images (**b**) from a cardiac CTA in an infant with congenital heart disease. The images show a single coronary artery arising from the left sinotubular junction well above the coronary sinus. The anatomy of the right and left coronary arteries is shown with a prepulmonary course of the RCA as well as the origins of the left anterior descending artery (LAD) and the circumflex artery (CX)

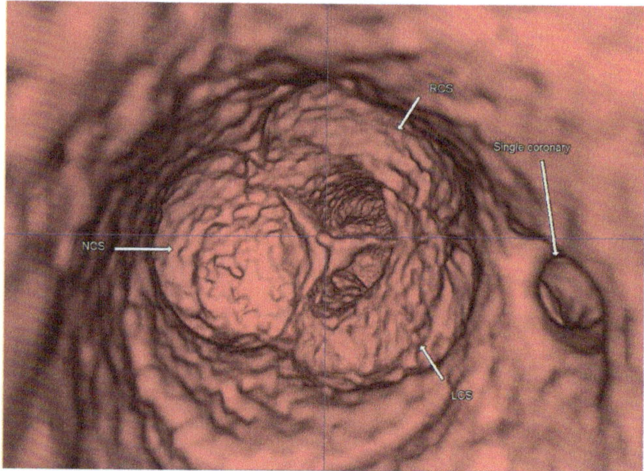

Fig. 3.10 Intraluminal 3D reconstruction from a cardiac CTA in an infant with known congenital heart disease. The image shows a single coronary artery arising from the left sinotubular junction well above the left coronary sinus (LCS). Right, left, and non- (RCS, LCS, NCS) coronary sinuses are also shown with no coronary artery origins

3.2.5 Right Coronary Artery Origin from the Left Coronary Sinus

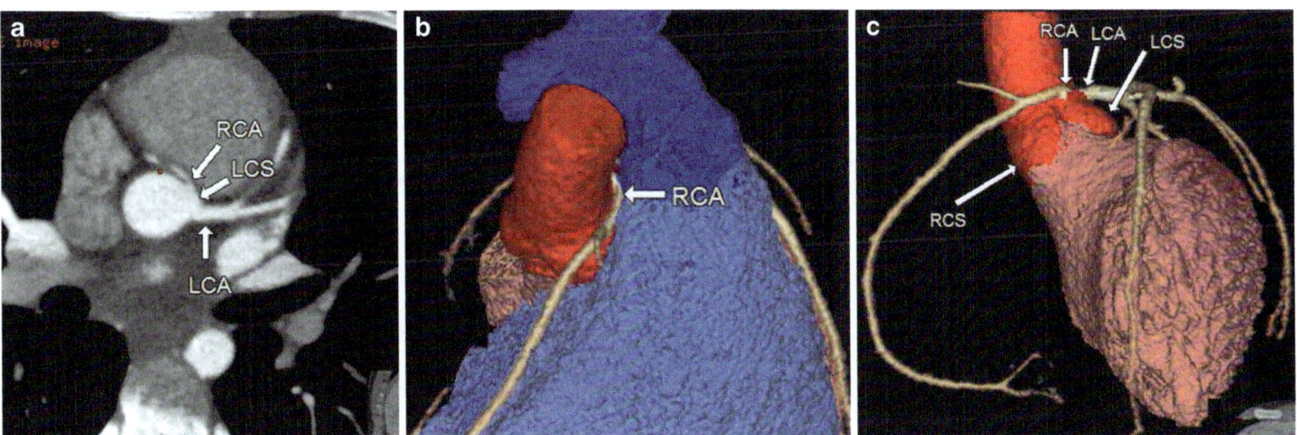

Fig. 3.11 MIP (**a**) and 3D color-coded images (**b, c**) from a cardiac CTA in a child. The images show an anomalous origin of the right coronary artery (RCA) from the left coronary sinus (LCS). In this case the course of the proximal right coronary artery was intramural, and the origin of the RCA was slit-like and diagonally oriented. The origin of the left coronary artery (LCA) was normal

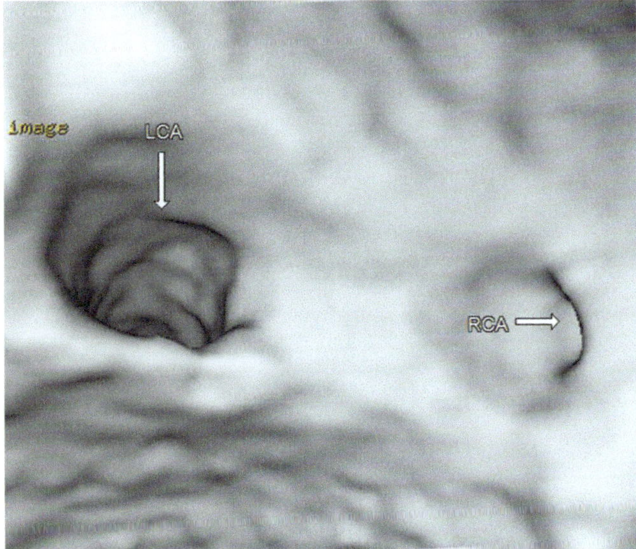

Fig. 3.12 Intraluminal 3D reconstruction from a cardiac CTA in a child showing the slit-like look and diagonal orientation of the right coronary artery (RCA). Notice the normal origin of the left coronary artery (LCA)

3.2.6   Left Coronary Artery Origin from the Right Coronary Sinus

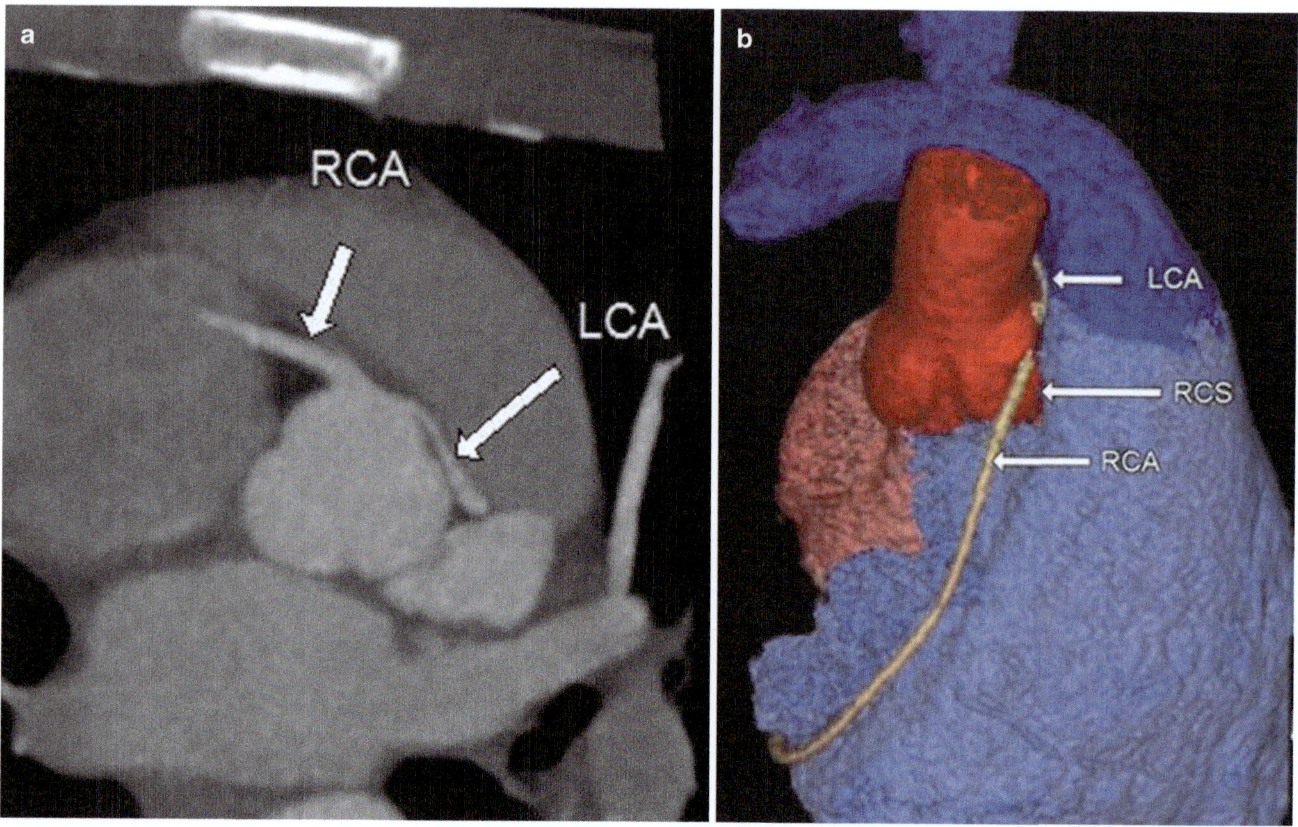

Fig. 3.13 MIP (**a**) and 3D color-coded images (**b**) from a cardiac CTA in a child. The images show an anomalous origin of the left cardiac artery (LCA) from the right coronary sinus (RCS). In this case the course of the proximal left coronary artery (LCA) was intramural, and its origin was slit-like and diagonally oriented. The origin of the right coronary artery (RCA) was normal

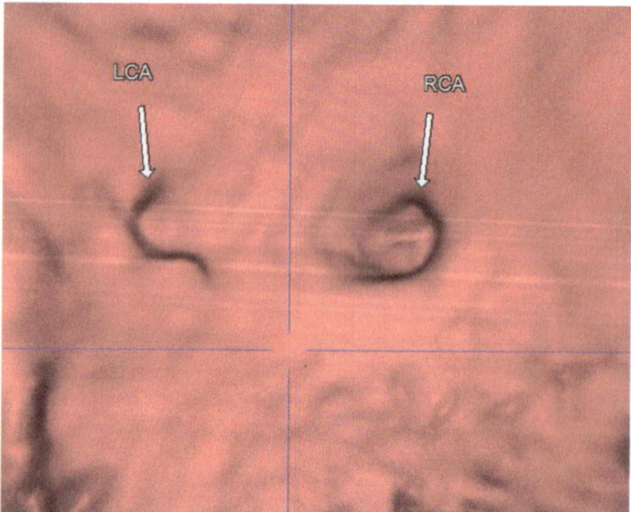

Fig. 3.14 Intraluminal 3D reconstruction from a cardiac CTA in a child showing the slit-like look and diagonal orientation of the left coronary artery (LCA). Notice the normal origin of the right coronary artery (RCA)

3.2.7   Right and Left Coronary Origin from Non-coronary Sinus

An anomalous left coronary artery arising from the pulmonary artery (ALCAPA) is a relatively rare anomaly in which the left coronary artery arises from the pulmonary artery instead of from the aorta. This anomaly can result in significant myocardial ischemia and infarction. This is typically caused by a coronary steal syndrome in which the flow in the higher pressure anomalous coronary artery is toward the lower pressure pulmonary artery, essentially "stealing" blood from the heart. Although it is more common for the left coronary artery to arise from the pulmonary artery, the right coronary artery can also arise from the pulmonary artery (ARCAPA) with the same physiologic flow from high to low pressure systems taking place.

There may normally be as many as four separate ostia of coronary arteries arising from the coronary sinuses. The most common anomaly is for the left anterior descending artery (LAD) and the circumflex artery (CX) to have separate origins from the left coronary sinus. A duplicated LAD from the right coronary sinus may also have a separate ostial opening.

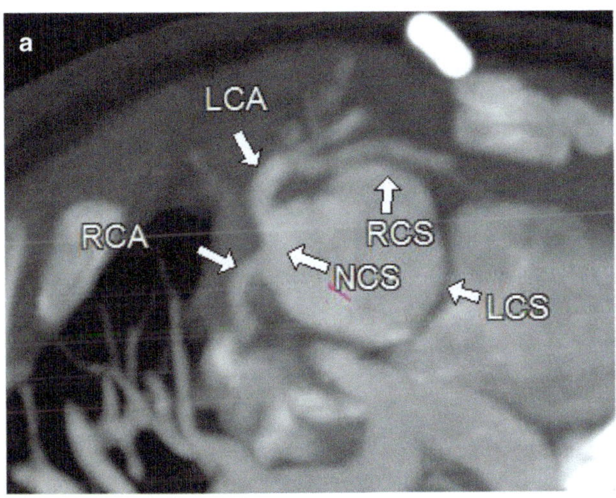

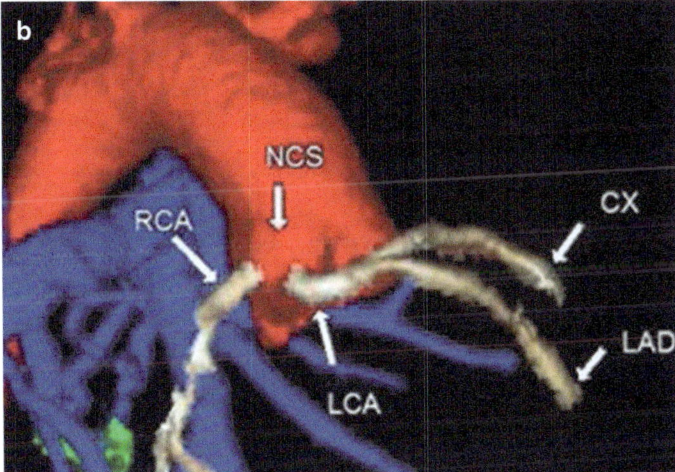

Fig. 3.15 MIP (**a**) and 3D color-coded images (**b**, **c**) from a cardiac CTA in an infant with congenital heart disease. The images show the anomalous origins of both the right and left (RCA and LCA) coronary arteries from the non-coronary sinus (NCS). Notice that there are no coronary arteries arising from the left and right coronary sinuses (LCS, RCS)

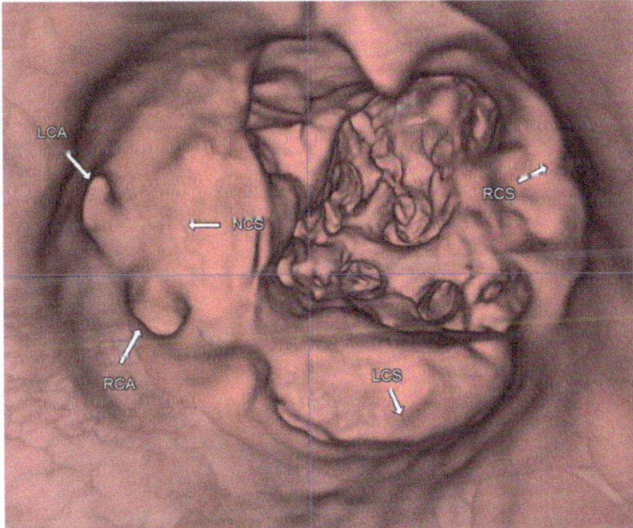

Fig. 3.16 Intraluminal 3D reconstruction from a cardiac CTA in an infant with known congenital heart disease. The image shows both the right and left (RCA and LCA) coronary arteries arising from the non-coronary sinus (NCS). Notice that there are no coronary arteries arising from the left and right coronary sinuses (LCS, RCS)

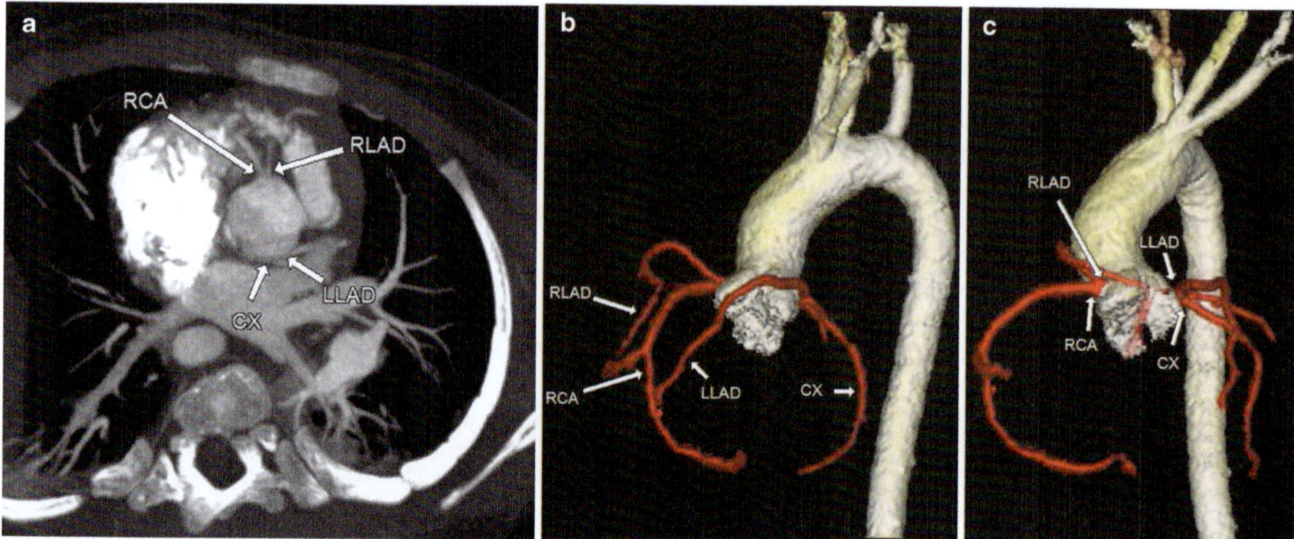

Fig. 3.17 MIP (**a**) and 3D color-coded images (**b, c**) from a cardiac CTA in an infant. The images show two coronary artery origins from both the right and left coronary sinuses. Notice that a duplicated left arterial descending artery (LAD) is seen, and the right sides of the LAD (RLAD) have a separate origin from the right cardiac artery (RCA) off the right coronary sinus (RCS). In addition, the circumflex (CX) and left LAD (LLAD) arteries have separate origins from the left coronary sinus (LCS)

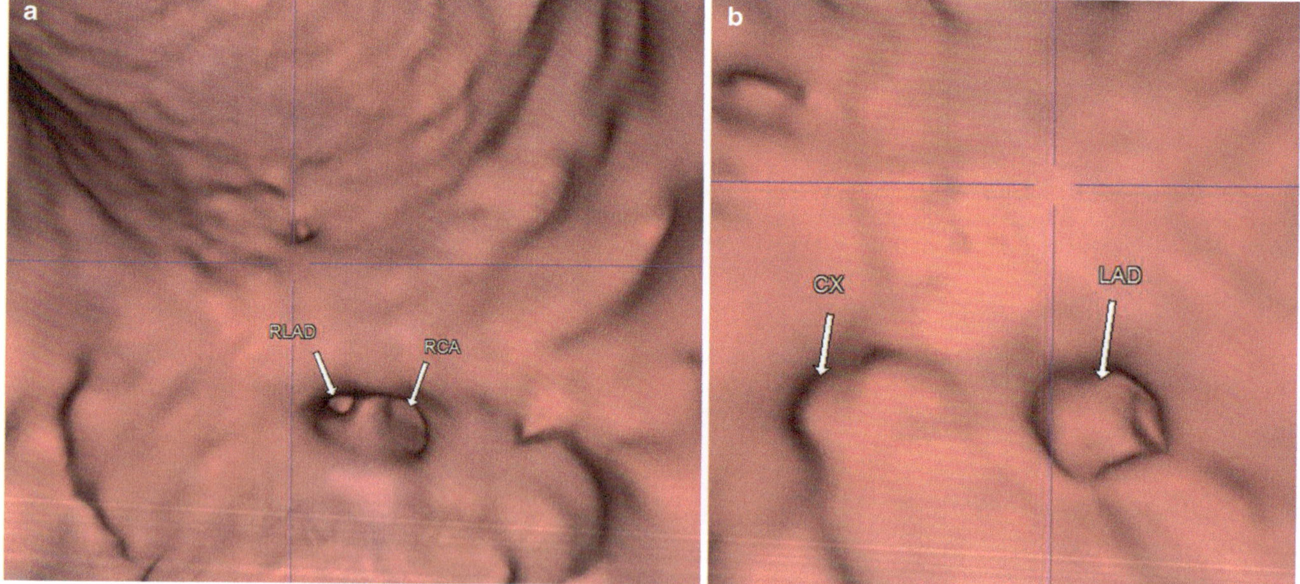

Fig. 3.18 Intraluminal 3D reconstruction images from a cardiac CTA in an infant with the right coronary sinus (RCS) (**a**) and the left coronary sinus (LCS) (**b**). The images show a duplicated anterior descending artery showing a separate origin of the RLAD from the right coronary sinus (RCS). In addition, the circumflex artery (CX) and the left arterial descending artery (LAD) have separate origins from the LCS

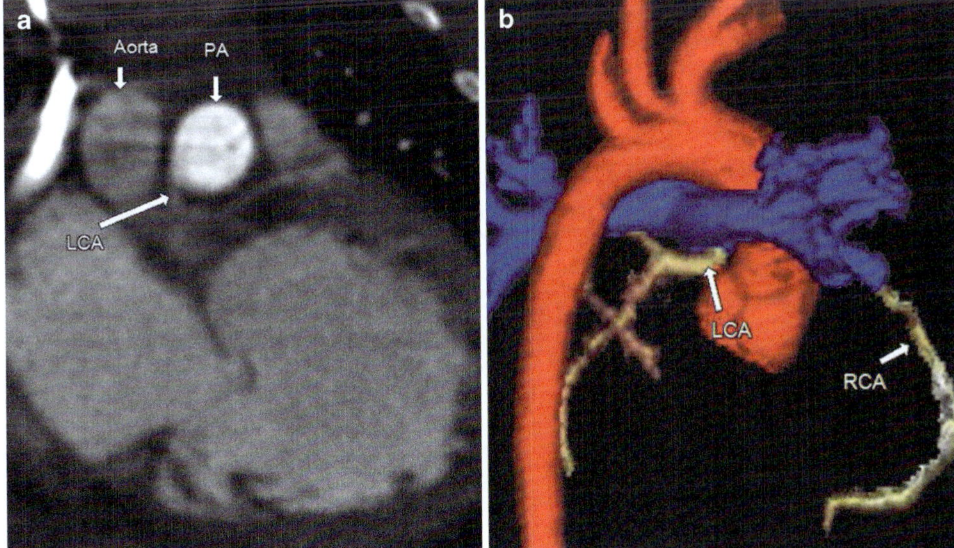

Fig. 3.19 MIP (**a**) and 3D color-coded images (**b**) from a cardiac CTA in an infant showing the left coronary artery (LCA) arising from the inferior right main pulmonary artery (MPA) instead of the aorta in a patient with ALCAPA. The right coronary artery (RCA) has a normal origin from the right coronary sinus (RCS)

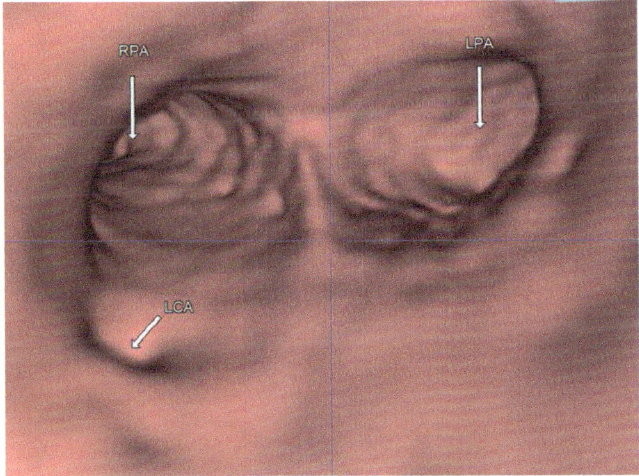

Fig. 3.20 Intraluminal 3D reconstruction from a cardiac CTA in an infant showing the origin of the left coronary artery (LCA) from the main pulmonary artery (MPA). Notice the bifurcation of the MPA into the right and left main pulmonary arteries (RPA, LPA)

3.3 Anomalous Left (or Right) Coronary Artery Arising from the Pulmonary Arteries (ALCAPA and ARCAPA)

Juxta-commissural origins of the coronary arteries should be described, especially in cases of myocardial ischemia or potential translocation of the coronary artery. Previous studies have shown that the right coronary artery origin is closer to the aortic commissures, especially between the right and left coronary sinuses.

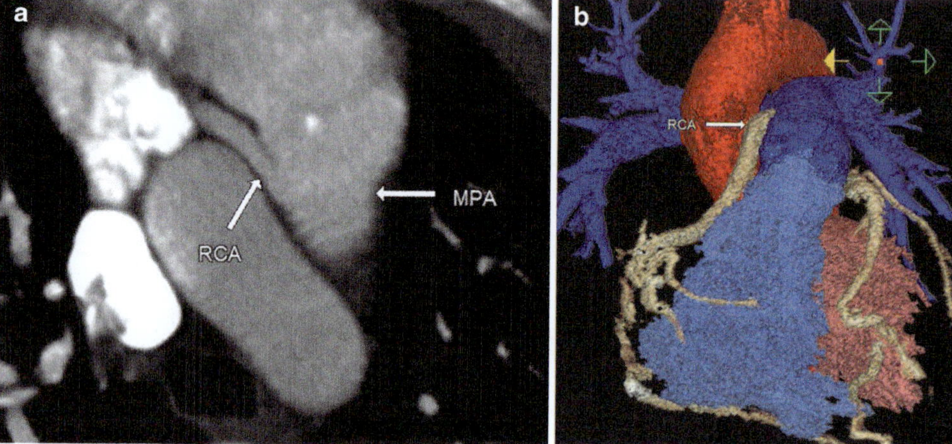

Fig. 3.21 MIP (**a**) and 3D color-coded images (**b**) from a cardiac CTA in an infant showing the right coronary artery (RCA) arising from the right side of the main pulmonary artery (MPA, *blue*) instead of the aorta in a patient with ARCAPA. The left coronary artery (LCA) had a normal origin from the left coronary sinus (LCS)

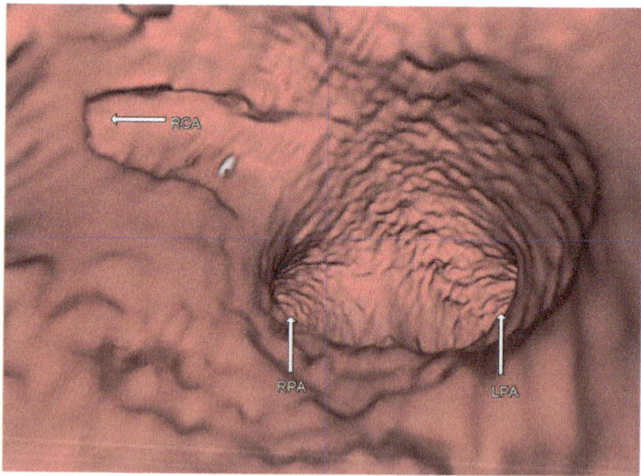

Fig. 3.22 Intraluminal 3D reconstruction from a cardiac CTA in an infant showing the origin of the right coronary artery (RCA) from the main pulmonary artery (MPA). Notice the bifurcation of the MPA into the right and left main pulmonary arteries (RPA, LPA)

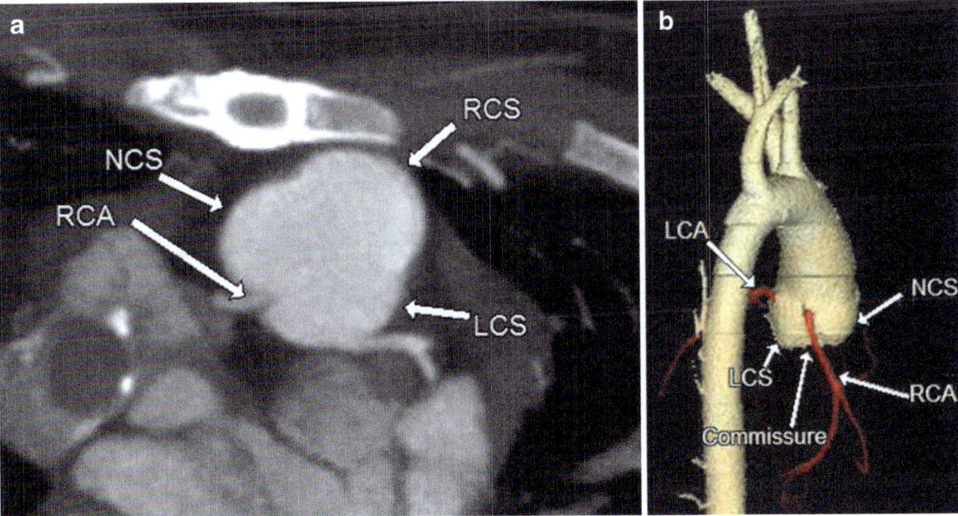

Fig. 3.23 MIP (**a**) and 3D color-coded images (**b**) from a cardiac CTA in an infant showing the right coronary artery (RCA) arising from just above or on the commissure between the left and non-coronary sinuses (LCS, NCS). The left coronary artery (LCA) arises normally from the left coronary sinus (LCS)

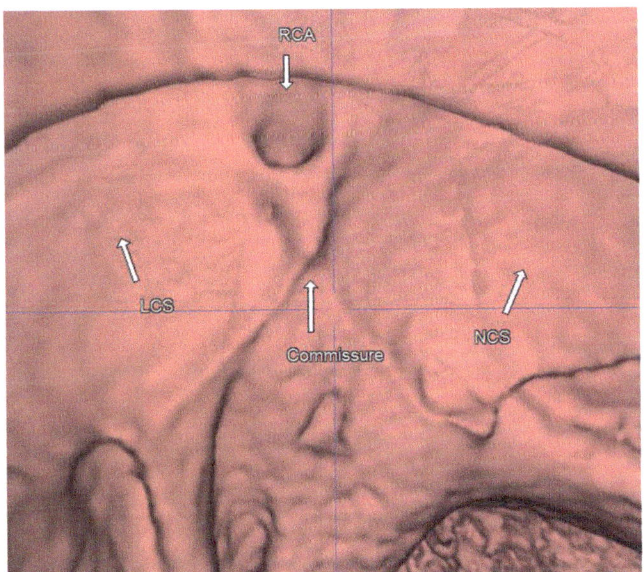

Fig. 3.24 Intraluminal 3D reconstruction from a cardiac CTA in a child shows the right coronary artery (RCA) arising from just above or on the commissure between the left and non-coronary sinuses (LCS, NCS)

Suggested Reading

Cacici G, Angelini P. Unusual case of single coronary artery: questions of methods and basic concepts. Ital Heart J. 2005;6:345–7.

Chiu IS, Anderson RH. Can we better understand the known variations in coronary arterial anatomy? Ann Thorac Surg. 2012;94:1751–60.

Elbadawi A, Baig B, Elgendy IY, Alotaki E, Mohamed AH, Barssoum K, et al. Single coronary artery anomaly: a case report and review of literature. Cardiol Ther. 2018;7:119–23.

Joshi SD, Joshi SS, Athavale SA. Origins of the coronary arteries and their significance. Clinics (Sao Paulo). 2010;65:79–84.

Venturini E, Magni L. Single coronary artery from the right sinus of Valsalva. Heart Int. 2011;6:e5.

Young PM, Gerber TC, Williamson EE, Julsrud PR, Herfkens RJ. Cardiac imaging: part 2, normal, variant, and anomalous configurations of the coronary vasculature. Am J Roentgenol. 2011;197:816–26.

Coronary artery origins can be altered in appearance in patients with congenital heart disease. Recognizing the type of congenital heart disease is key to understanding some predictable variations in the coronary artery origins.

4.1 Aortic Atresia

Aortic atresia with a hypoplastic ascending aorta can have an unusual appearance. The coronary origins are typically normal, but the ascending aorta is so small that it is often similar in size to the coronary arteries (Fig. 4.1).

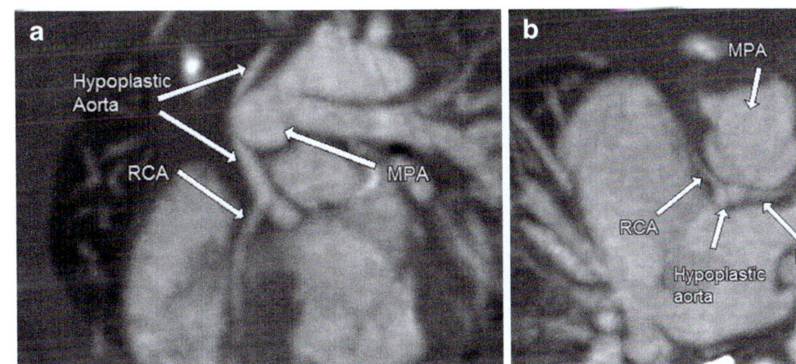

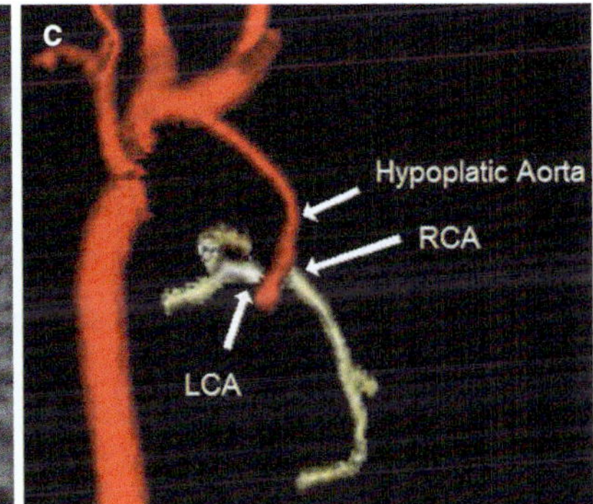

Fig. 4.1 (a–c) Oblique coronal (a) and axial (b) maximum intensity projection (MIP) images as well as a volume-rendered 3D image (c) demonstrating the anatomy in a patient with aortic atresia and marked hypoplasia of the ascending aorta. Notice that the right (RCA) and left (LCA) coronary arteries arise from where you would expect the right and left coronary sinuses to be. The sinuses are also hypoplastic

R. R. Richardson, *Atlas of Pediatric CTA of Coronary Artery Anomalies*, https://doi.org/10.1007/978-3-030-28087-1_4

4.2   Truncus Arteriosus

Truncus arteriosus is a relatively rare congenital heart defect in which a single common vessel arises from the heart from the right and left ventricles instead of two vessels. The coronary origins in a patient with truncus arteriosus may vary, as the common truncal valve may have two, three, or four cusps. For the bicuspid and tricuspid valves the coronary origins typically follow the pattern of arising from the sinuses facing the pulmonary trunk. In a quadracuspid truncal valve the origin of the left coronary artery is often displaced posteriorly and to the right, since it wraps around a pulmonary sinus that is incorporated into the common trunk. Rarely, a coronary artery may arise from the pulmonary artery component of the truncal root. A single coronary artery also can be seen with truncus arteriosus (Fig. 4.2) [1–3].

4.3   Transposition of the Great Arteries

Transposition of the great arteries is the second most common most cyanotic congenital heart defect. It is seen when the aorta and pulmonary arteries are connected/transposed to the incorrect ventricle. Dextro-transposition (D-TGA) of the great arteries is more common than Levo or corrected type transposition (L-TGA) of the great vessels. The pattern for coronary artery origins in these patients is for the coronary arteries to arise from the sinuses that face the pulmonary artery (facing sinuses). There are some variations that do occur and are important for the surgeon to understand before performing an arterial switch procedure, since the coronaries will need to be translocated from one great vessel to the other. The more common variations are illustrated in this chapter (Fig. 4.3).

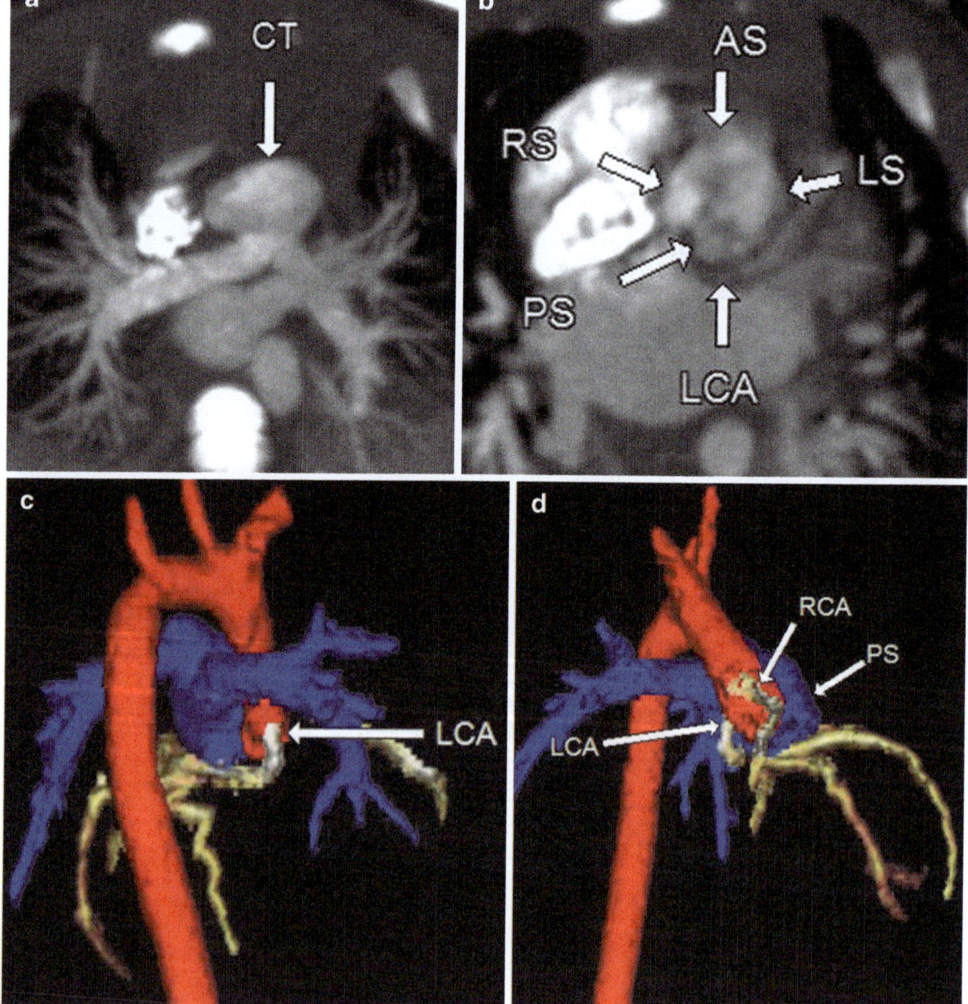

Fig. 4.2 (**a–d**) Axial MIP images (**a**, **b**) and volume-rendered 3D images (**c**, **d**) from a cardiac CTA in a patient with truncus arteriosus show the common trunk (CT) with a common origin of the aorta and pulmonary arteries. A quadracuspid valve is shown on the right with the right aortic sinus (RS), the anterior aortic sinus (AS), the left aortic sinus (LS), and a fourth sinus that is part of the pulmonary sinus (PS). Notice how the left coronary origin goes posteriorly around the pulmonary sinus from the right aortic sinus. The right coronary artery (RCA) comes off the anterior aortic sinus. This is a typical pattern seen with a quadracuspid valve in a patient with Truncus arteriosus

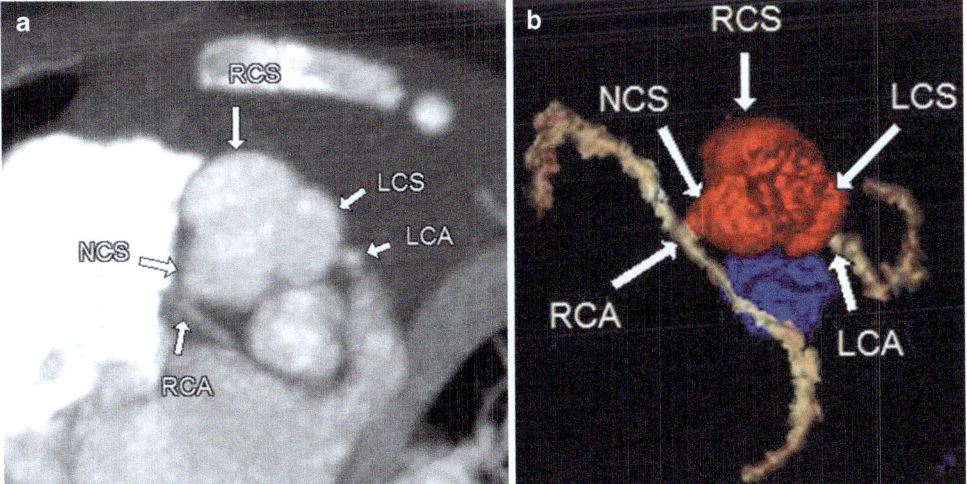

Fig. 4.3 MIP axial (**a**) and inferior view from a volume-rendered 3D color-coded image (**b**) from a cardiac CTA in an infant with D-TGA showing the typical pattern of coronary artery origins with the right coronary artery (RCA) arising from the noncoronary sinus (NCS) and the left coronary artery (LCA) arising from the left coronary sinus (LCS). Notice that there is no coronary artery arising from the right coronary sinus because it is not one of the two sinuses facing the pulmonary artery

Fig. 4.4 Intraluminal 3D (3 D) reconstruction (**a**) and lateral view from a volume-rendered 3-D image (**b**) from a cardiac CTA in an infant with known D-TGA again shows the typical pattern of coronary artery origins with the right coronary artery (RCA) arising from the noncoronary sinus (NCS) and the left coronary artery (LCA) arising from the left coronary sinus (LCS). Notice that there is no coronary artery arising from the right coronary sinus (RCS) because it is not one of the two sinuses facing the pulmonary artery

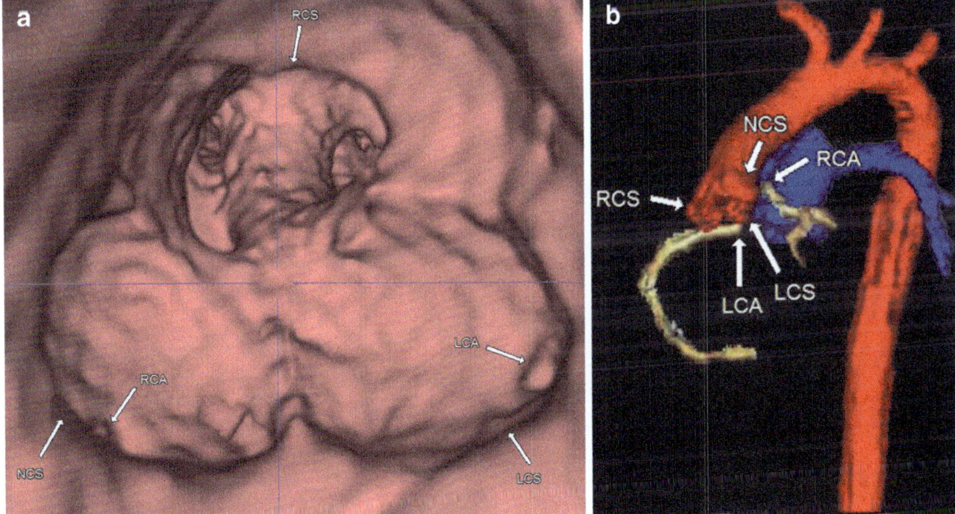

4.4   Patterns of Coronary Anomalies in Transposition of the Great Arteries

Normally the coronary arteries arise from the sinuses facing the pulmonary artery. In patients with transposition of the great arteries this is also the case but because the great vessels are transposed the coronaries typically arise from the left and non-coronary sinuses instead of the right and left coronary sinuses. We will show the patterns of coronary artery anomalies seen in transposition of the great arteries.

4.5   Aortic Root Rotation Causing Interarterial Origin

Another common occurrence in patients with congenital heart disease and especially common in patients with tetralogy of Fallot, is the appearance of significant clockwise rotation of the aortic root. This rotation causes the right coronary sinus to be in a left anterior position so that the origin of the right coronary right coronary artery is to the left of the midline. In patients with pulmonic atresia this is not a problem, but when a pulmonic homograft is placed, it can cause narrowing and possible obstruction at the origin of the right coronary artery (Figs. 4.14 and 4.15) [6].

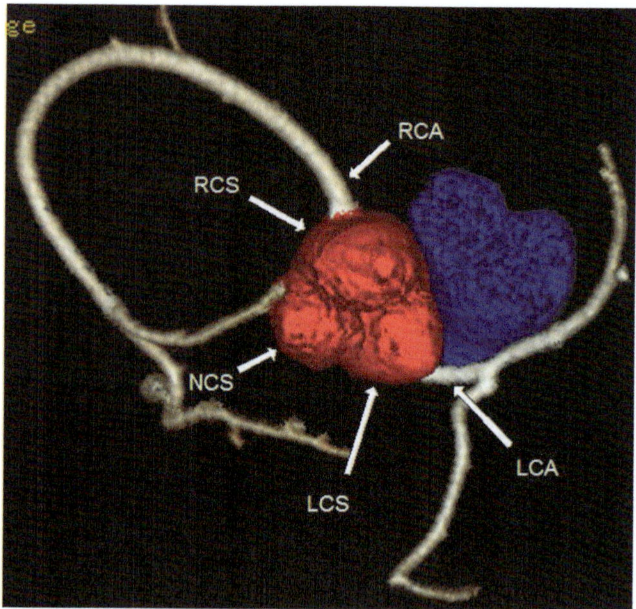

Fig. 4.5 Single inferior view volume-rendered 3D image from a cardiac CTA in an infant showing the normal coronary artery origins with the right coronary artery (RCA) arising from the right coronary sinus (RCS) and the left coronary artery (LCA) arising from the left coronary sinus (LCS). Notice that the coronary arteries arise from the sinus facing the pulmonary artery so that the noncoronary sinus has no coronary artery origin

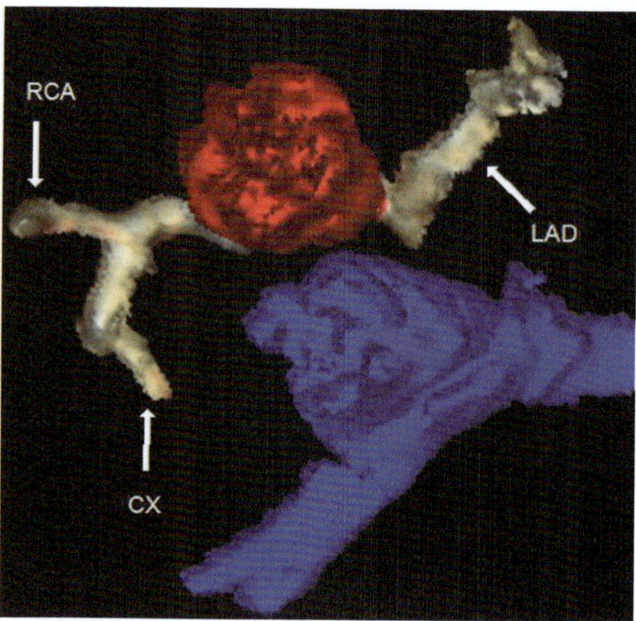

Fig. 4.7 Single inferior view volume-rendered 3D image from a cardiac CTA in an infant with D-TGA shows a slight variation in the pattern, with the left anterior descending artery (LAD) arising from the left coronary sinus and the right coronary artery arising from the noncoronary sinus (NCS). Notice that circumflex (CX) coronary artery arises from the RCA

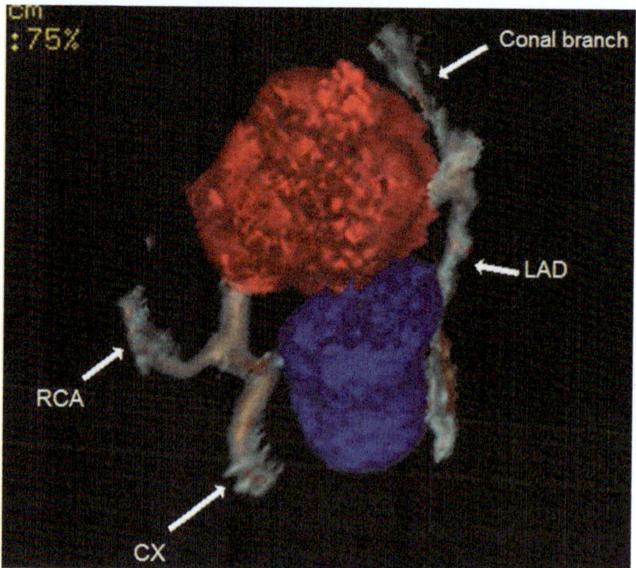

Fig. 4.6 Single inferior view volume-rendered 3D image from a cardiac CTA in an infant with D-TGA again shows the typical pattern in which the left coronary artery (LCA) arises from the left coronary sinus (LCS) and then branches into the left anterior descending artery (LAD) and circumflex coronary artery (CX) and the right coronary artery (RCA) arises from the noncoronary sinus (NCS)

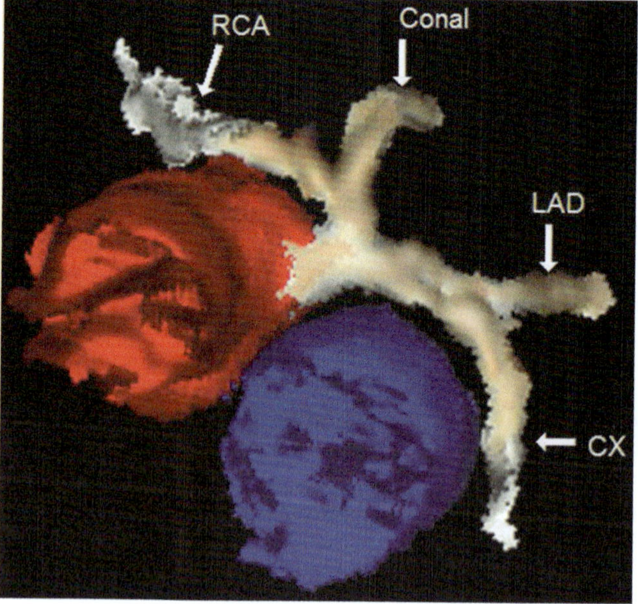

Fig. 4.8 Single inferior view volume-rendered 3D image from a cardiac CTA in an infant with D-TGA showing the right coronary artery (RCA), left anterior descending artery (LAD), and circumflex artery (CX), all arising from the left-sided single coronary artery. Notice that the RCA courses anterior to the aorta. A prominent conal branch is also noted

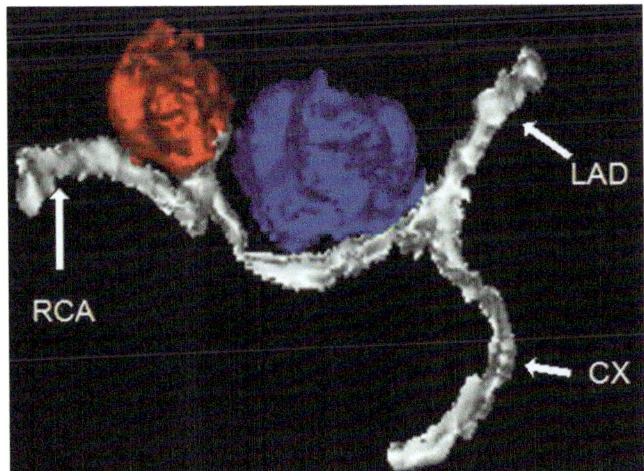

Fig. 4.9 Single inferior view volume-rendered 3D image from a cardiac CTA in an infant with D-TGA shows another single coronary artery arising from the left coronary sinus. However, in this example the left coronary artery (LCA) courses posterior to the pulmonary artery before branching into the left anterior descending artery (LAD) and the circumflex artery (CX). The right coronary artery (RCA) courses posterior to the aorta

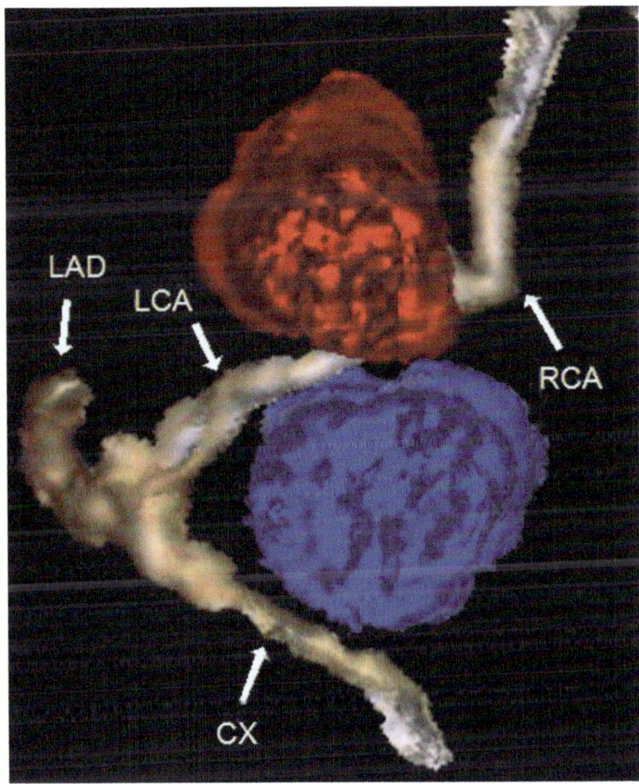

Fig. 4.10 Single inferior view volume-rendered 3D image from a cardiac CTA in an infant with D-TGA shows an inverted pattern with the left coronary artery (LCA) coming off the noncoronary sinus (NCS) and the right coronary artery (RCA) coming off the left coronary sinus (LCS). This is seen in patients with situs anomalies in addition to those with transposition of the great vessels

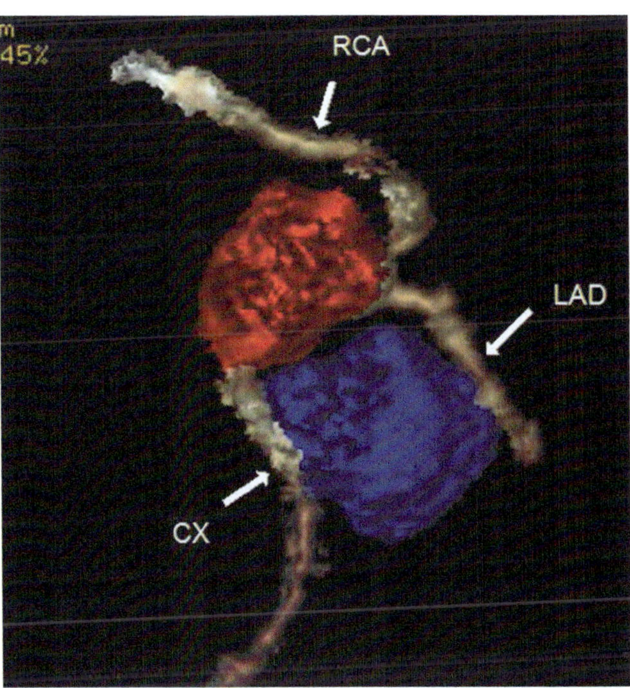

Fig. 4.11 Single inferior view volume-rendered 3D image from a cardiac CTA in an infant with D-TGA shows the inversion of the right coronary artery (RCA) and the circumflex artery (CX), with the RCA arising from the left coronary sinus and the CX arising from the noncoronary sinus. Notice that the left anterior descending artery (LAD) and the RCA have a common origin

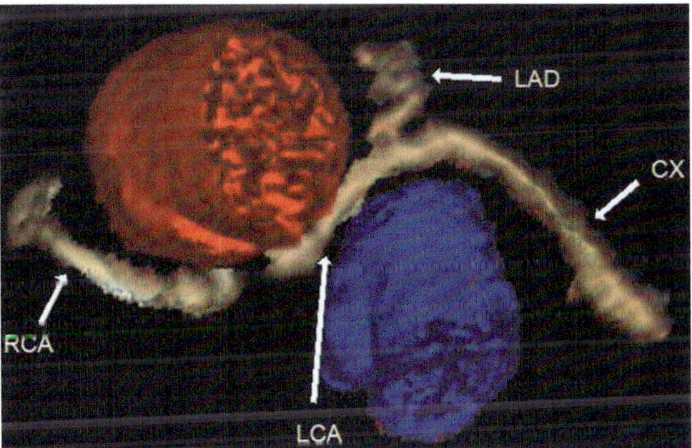

Fig. 4.12 Single inferior view volume-rendered 3D image from a cardiac CTA in an infant with D-TGA shows an interarterial course of the proximal left anterior descending artery (LAD). This may be an intramural course of the left main coronary artery. Otherwise the anatomy is typical, with the right coronary artery (RCA) arising from the noncoronary sinus (NCS) and normal bifurcation of the left anterior descending artery (LAD) and the circumflex artery (CX)

Fig. 4.13 (**a, b**) Two MIP images from a cardiac CTA in an infant with D-TGA status post-arterial switch procedures with translocation of the coronary arteries. The pulmonary artery is now anterior to the aorta posterior, and the right and left coronary arteries (RCA, LCA) come off the anterior right and left coronary sinuses [4, 5]

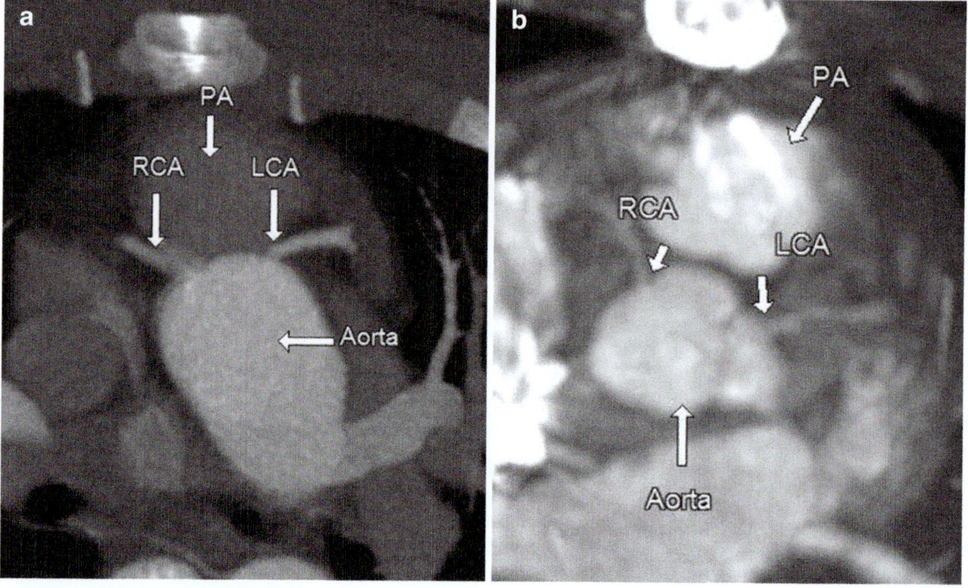

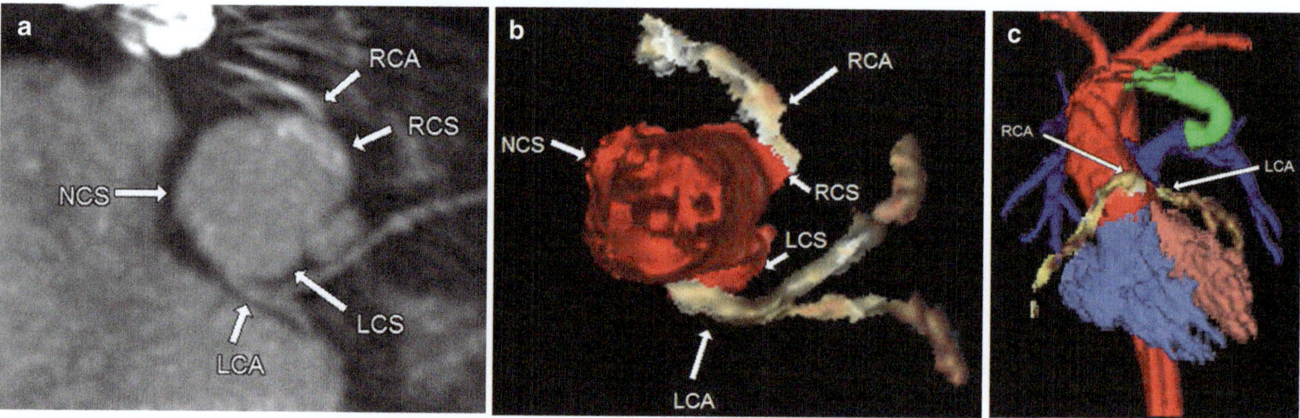

Fig. 4.14 MIP axial (**a**), inferior (**b**), and frontal (**c**) views from volume-rendered 3D images in a patient with Tetralogy of Fallot and pulmonic atresia show clockwise rotation of the aortic root with the right coronary sinus (RCS) in the left anterior position, and the origin of the right coronary artery (RCA) from the RCS is left-sided. The left coronary artery (LCA) arises in the posterior right position from the rotated left coronary sinus (LCS). This position of the origin of the RCA is not currently a problem because there is complete pulmonic atresia, with the flow to the pulmonary arteries (*blue*) forming a PDA (*green*) arising from the left brachiocephalic artery

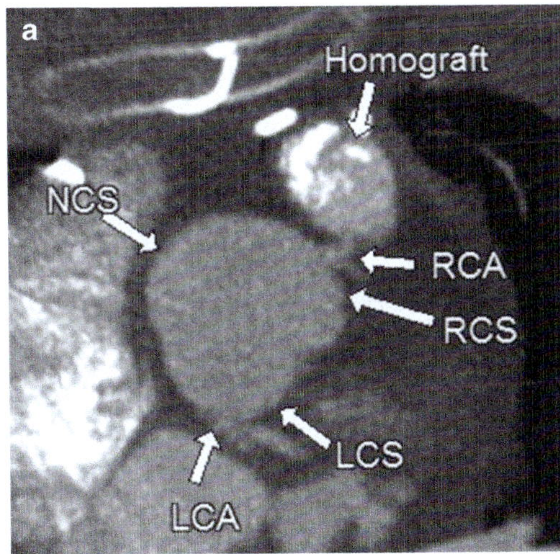
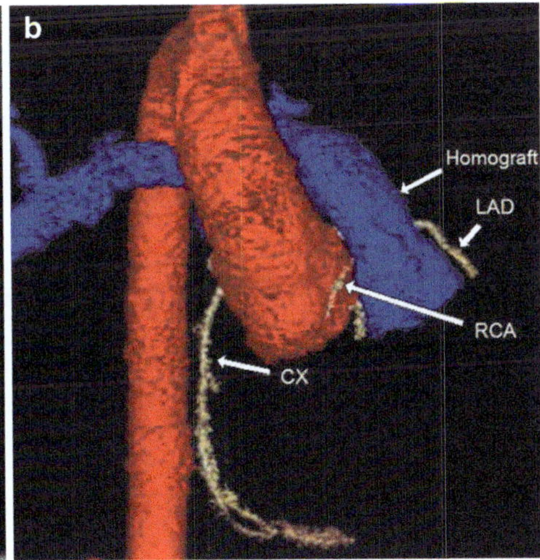

Fig. 4.15 MIP axial (**a**) and volume-rendered 3D images (**b**) from a cardiac CTA in a teenage patient who had Tetralogy of Fallot repair with a pulmonary homograft in place. Notice the severe clockwise rotation of the aortic root with the right coronary sinus (RCS) in the left anterior position and the origin of the right coronary artery (RCA) between the pulmonary homograft and the ascending aorta. The RCA is now hypoplastic from chronic compression at its origin. The aortic root rotation is further shown by the anterior right position of the noncoronary sinus (NCS) and the posterior right position of the left coronary sinus (LCS). The origin of the left coronary artery (LCA) is posterior and to the left

References

1. Shrivastava S, Edwards JE. Coronary arterial origin in persistent truncus arteriosus. Circulation. 1977;55:551–4.
2. de la Cruz MV, Cayre R, Angelini P, Noriega-Ramos N, Sadowinski S. Coronary arteries in truncus arteriosus. Am J Cardiol. 1990;66:1482–6.
3. Rodríguez H, Montero H, Fernández A, Guzman A, Sessa TD. Surgical correction of truncus arteriosus with unusual origin of the right coronary artery. World J Pediatr Congenit Heart Surg. 2016;7:407–10.
4. Massoudy P, Baltalarli A, de Leval MR, Cook A, Neudorf U, Derrick G, et al. Anatomic variability in coronary arterial distribution with regard to the arterial switch procedure. Circulation. 2002;106:1980–4.
5. Scognamiglio G, Li W. Arterial switch operation for transposition of great arteries: late results in adult patients. ICFJ. 2015;1:8. https://doi.org/10.17987/icfj.v1i1.13.
6. Tretter JT, Mori S, Saremi F, Chikkabyrappa S, Thomas K, Bu F, et al. Variations in rotation of the aortic root and membranous septum with implications for transcatheter valve implantation. Heart. 2018;104:999–1005.

There are a wide range of variations in the course of the coronary arteries. An understanding of the common anomalous courses of the coronaries is helpful when looking at infants and children, in whom the size of the coronary arteries is significantly smaller than those in adults. Anomalies and variations of the course of the coronaries are often seen when their origin is from the opposite sinus. Common pathways for these anomalies of origin are interarterial, prepulmonary, retro- or circum-aortic, trans-septal, and retrocardiac. The interarterial course may be intramural or within the wall of the aorta. This can have adverse clinical outcomes.

5.1 Prepulmonary

See Figs. 5.1, 5.2, 5.3, and 5.4.

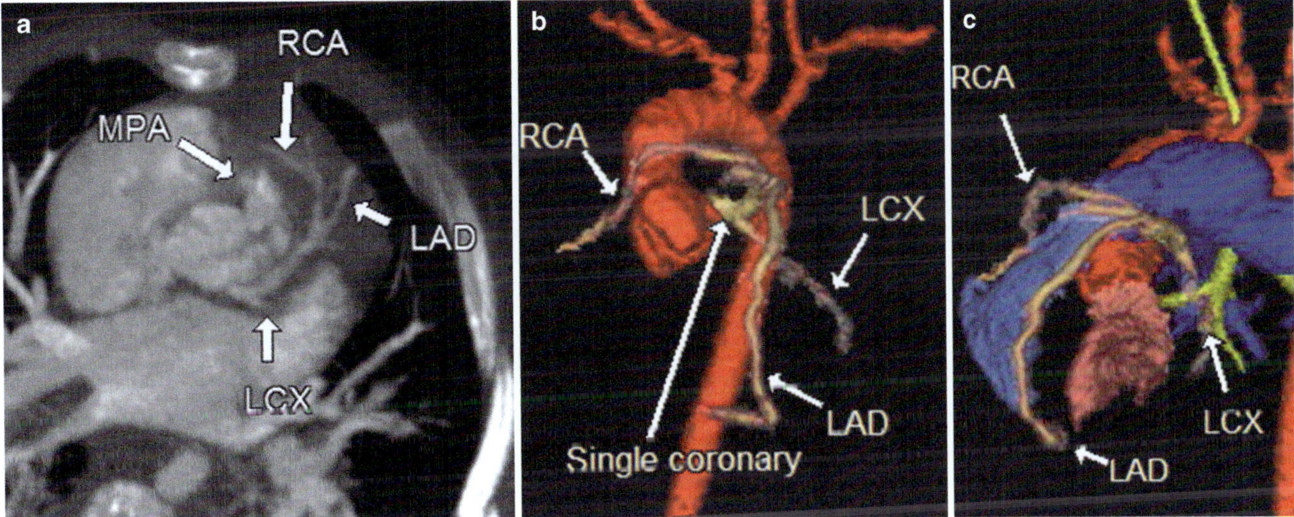

Fig. 5.1 Axial maximum intensity projection (MIP) (a) and frontal (b) and left (c) lateral 3D images from a cardiac computed tomography angiography (CTA) in an infant showing a single left coronary artery (LCA) arising from the left coronary sinus. The right coronary artery (RCA) courses from left to right in front of the main pulmonary artery (MPA, *blue*). This is referred to as a prepulmonary course. This can be significant if a pulmonary homograft needs to be placed, since the coronary artery would be in the path where dissection would take place. Notice the normal course of the LCA and the circumflex (LCX) and left anterior descending (LAD) coronary arteries

© Springer Nature Switzerland AG 2020
R. R. Richardson, *Atlas of Pediatric CTA of Coronary Artery Anomalies*, https://doi.org/10.1007/978-3-030-28087-1_5

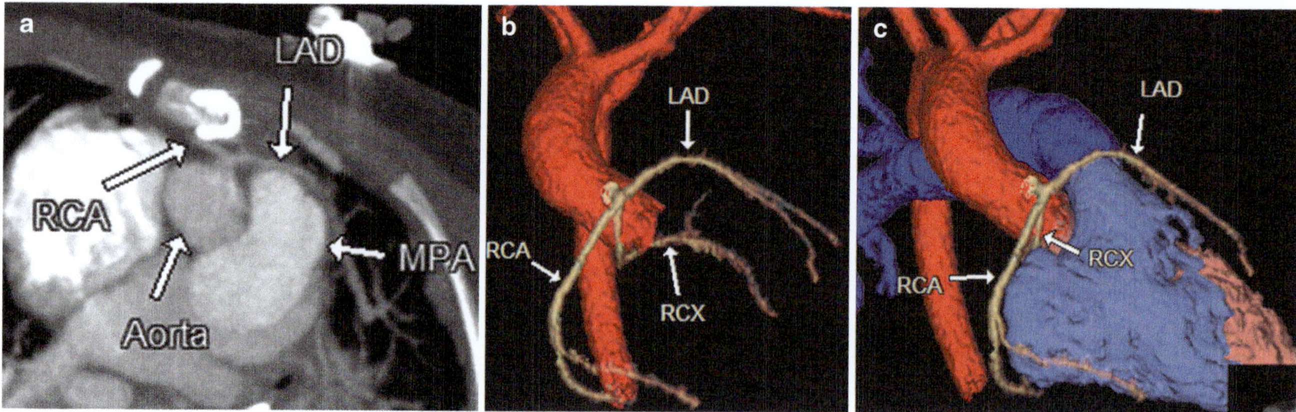

Fig. 5.2 Axial MIP (**a**) and frontal and left lateral third images (**b, c**) from a cardiac CTA in an infant show a single right coronary artery (RCA) arising from the right coronary sinus. The left anterior descending coronary artery (LAD) has a prepulmonary course from right to left in front of the main pulmonary artery (MPA, *blue*). Notice the circumaortic course of the right circumflex artery (RCX) from right to left and the normal course of the RCA

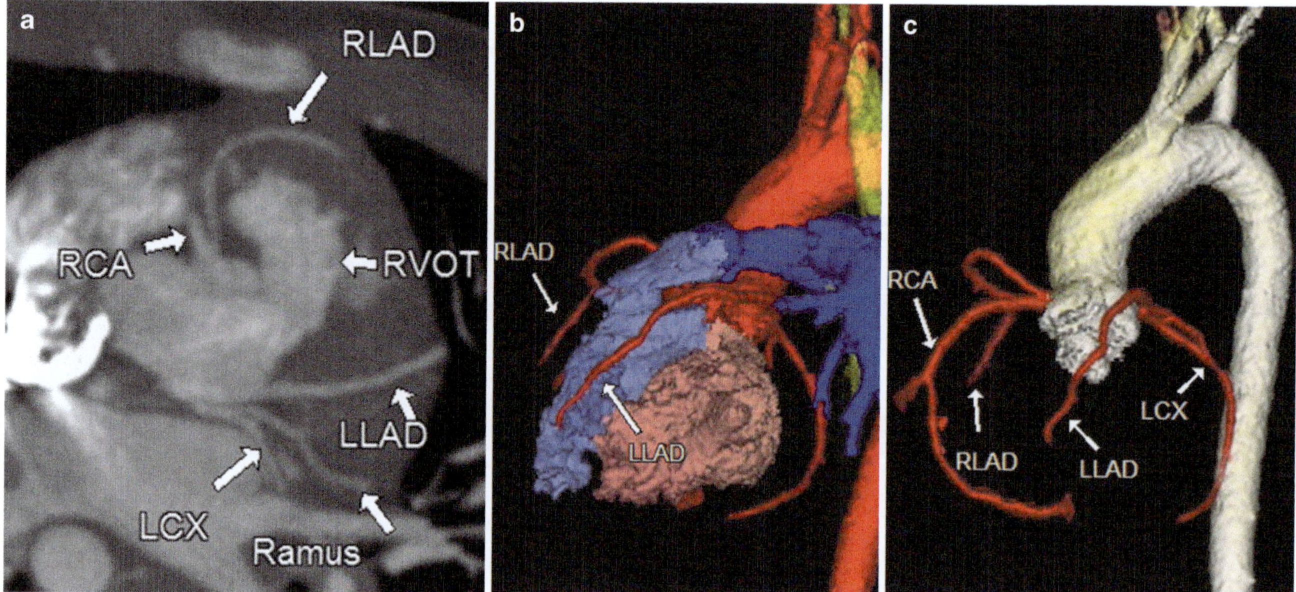

Fig. 5.3 Axial MIP (**a**) and lateral 3D images (**b, c**) from a cardiac CTA in an infant show a duplicated anterior descending coronary artery arising from the right coronary sinus and then coursing in front of the right ventricular outflow tract (*purple*). The right (RCA) and left (LCA) coronary arteries have a normal course with normal branching of the left anterior descending (LAD) and circumflex (LCX) arteries

5.2 Circumaortic

A circumaortic course of the coronary artery occurs when the right coronary arises from the left coronary sinus or when the left coronary or circumflex arises from the right coronary sinus and courses posterior to the aorta before reaching its normal position on the opposite side.

Fig. 5.4 Axial MIP (**a**) and lateral 3D images (**b**) from a cardiac CTA in an infant show a prominent conal branch arising from the right coronary sinus and then coursing in front of the right ventricular outflow tract (*purple*). The right (RCA) and left (LCA) coronary arteries have a normal course with normal branching of the left anterior descending (LAD) and circumflex (LCX) arteries

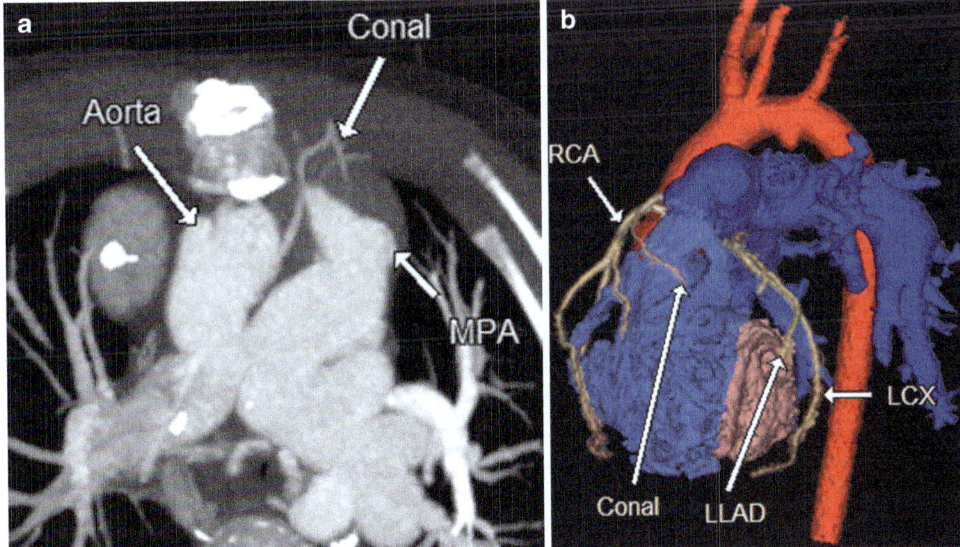

Fig. 5.5 Axial MIP (**a**) and frontal 3D images (**b**) from a cardiac CTA in an infant show a single right coronary artery (RCA) arising from the right coronary sinus. The left anterior descending coronary artery (LAD) has a prepulmonary course from right to left in front of the main pulmonary artery. The circumflex (RCX) artery has a circumaortic course from right to left, and there is a normal course of the RCA

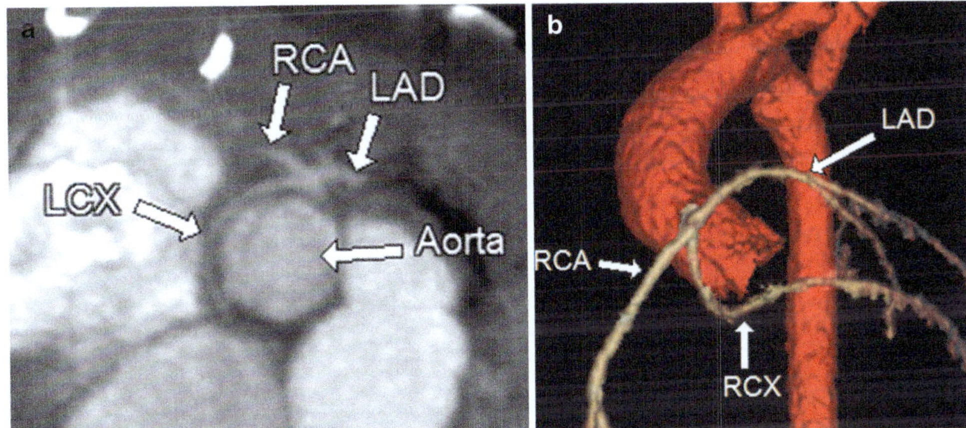

Fig. 5.6 Axial MIP (**A**) and lateral 3D images (**B**) from a cardiac CTA in an infant showing a single right coronary artery arising from the right coronary sinus. The left coronary artery (LCA) has a circumaortic course from right to left and then branches into the circumflex (LCX) and left anterior descending (LAD) arteries. There is a normal course of the right coronary artery (RCA)

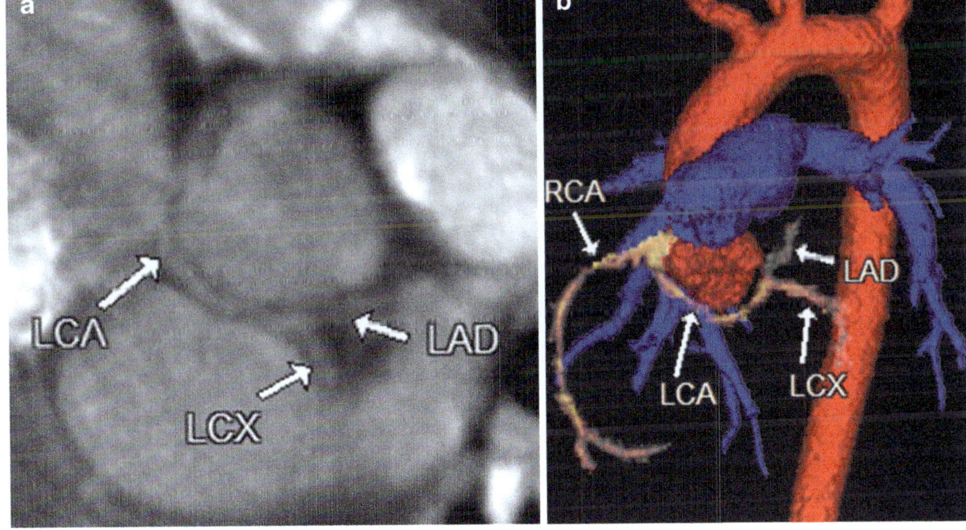

Fig. 5.7 Axial MIP (**a**) and lateral 3D images (**b**) from a cardiac CTA in a child show a single coronary artery arising from the left sinotubular junction. The right coronary artery (RCA) courses from left to right anterior to the aorta and then between the main pulmonary artery (MPA) and the aorta. This is an interarterial course. Notice that the branches of the left coronary artery have a normal course, dividing into circumflex (LCX) and left anterior descending (LAD) arteries

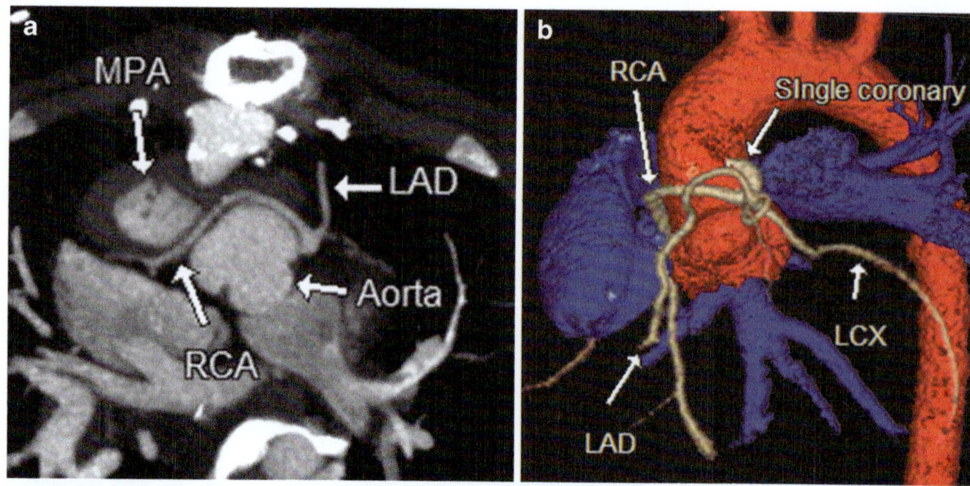

Fig. 5.8 Axial MIP (**a**) and lateral 3D images (**b**) from a cardiac CTA in a child show the left coronary artery (LCA) arising from the right coronary sinus. The LCA courses from right to left anterior to the aorta and then between the main pulmonary artery (MPA) and the aorta. The right coronary artery (RCA) has a normal course

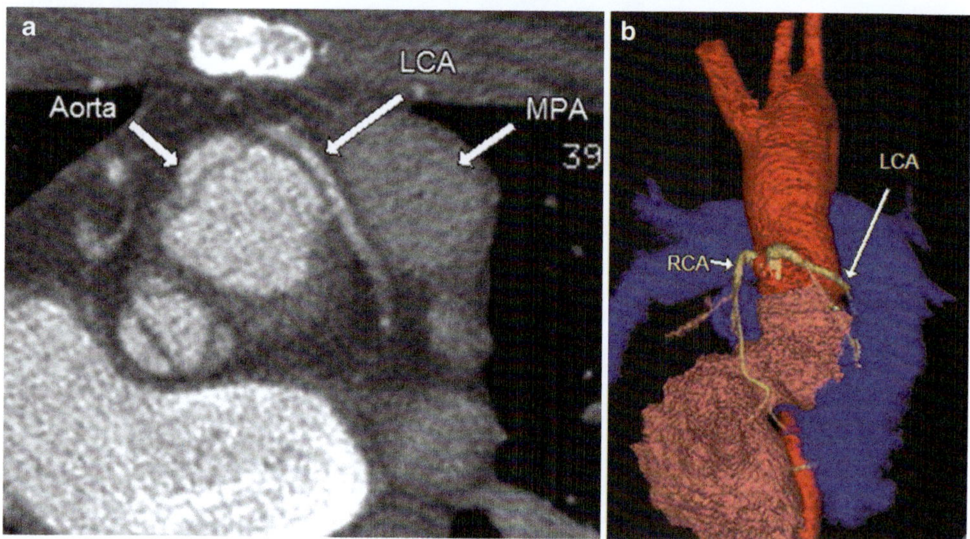

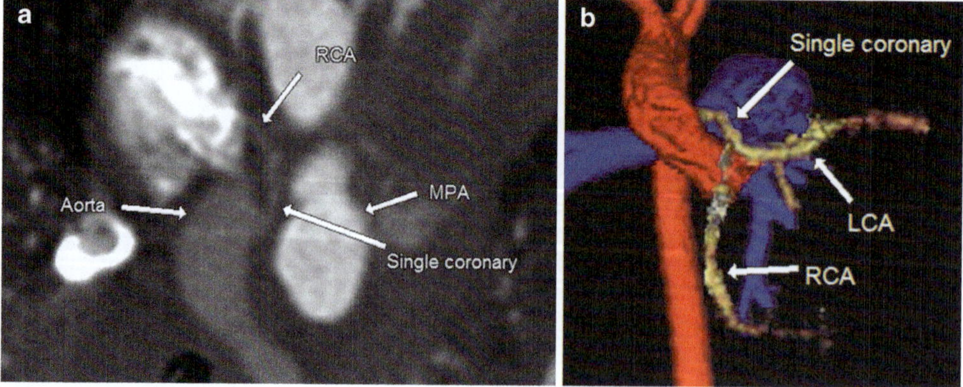

Fig. 5.9 Axial MIP (**a**) and lateral 3D images (**b**) from a cardiac CTA in an infant showing a single coronary artery arising from the left sinotubular junction. The proximal common coronary artery courses anteriorly between the main pulmonary artery (MPA) and the aorta (*red*). The right (RCA) and left (LCA) coronary arteries then branch, with a normal course of the RCA. Notice that the LCA courses under the MPA before branching

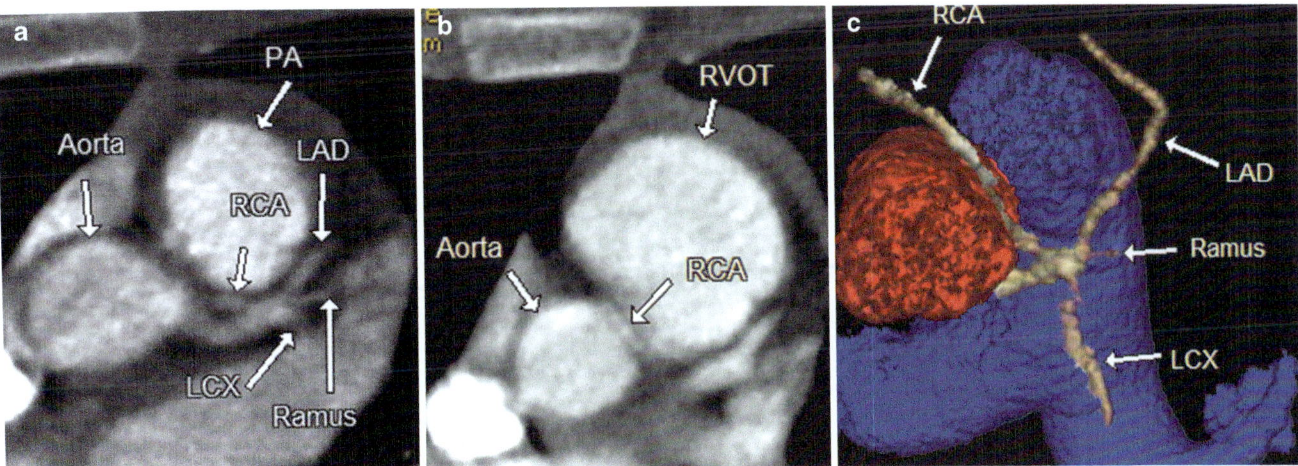

Fig. 5.10 Axial MIP images (**a**, **b**) and lateral 3D images (**c**) from a cardiac CTA in a child showing a single coronary artery arising from the left coronary sinus. The right coronary artery (RCA) arises from the proximal left coronary artery (LCA) and then courses from left to right between the main pulmonary artery (MPA) and the aorta. This is an interarterial course. Notice that the branches of the LCA have a normal course, dividing into circumflex (LCX) and left anterior descending (LAD) arteries

Fig. 5.11 Axial MIP (**a**) and lateral 3D images (**b**) from a cardiac CTA in a child showing the left coronary artery (LCA) arising from the right coronary sinus and then coursing from right to left between the main pulmonary artery (*blue*) and the aorta (*red*). There is narrowing of the proximal LCA, and the patient showed a 9-mm intramural course along the wall of the aorta before exiting into a normal course

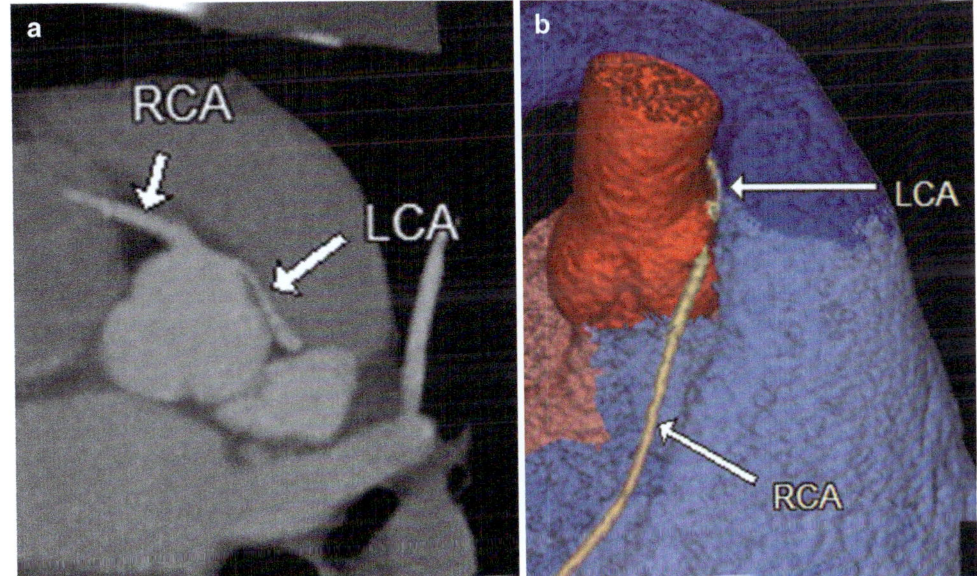

5.3 Intramural

Another possible anomaly for the coronaries when coursing from right to left or left to right is to go between the aorta and main pulmonary artery; this is referred to as Interarterial. An interarterial course may be intramural. An intramural course means that there is a portion of the coronary artery within the wall of the aorta. An intramural course increase is more predictive of an adverse outcome (Figs. 5.11, 5.12, 5.13, 5.14, 5.15, and 5.16).

Fig. 5.12 Two coronal images (**a**, **b**) from a cardiac CTA in a child showing side-to-side narrowing of the proximal left coronary artery (LCA); the patient showed a 9-mm intramural course along the wall of the aorta before exiting into a normal course. The increased height–width ratio of 2:1 correlates well with an intramural course. An interarterial course without an intramural segment typically has a 1:1 height-to-width ratio

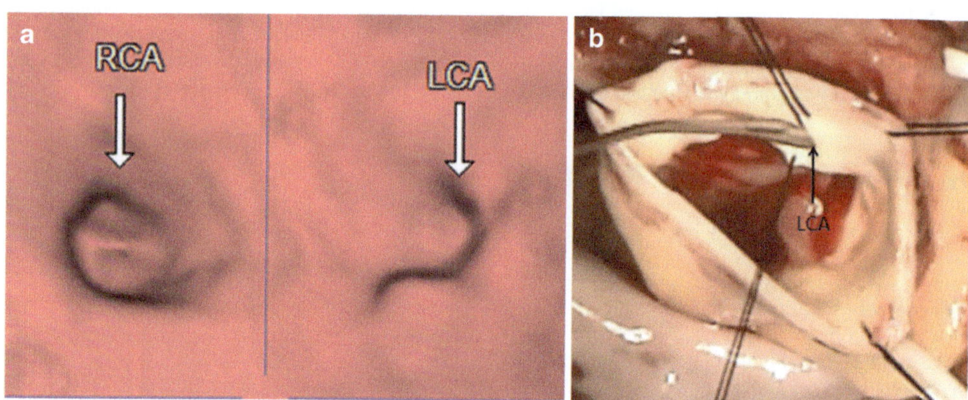

Fig. 5.13 Virtual angioscopy image (**a**) from a cardiac CTA of a child and intraoperative image (**b**). The left image shows the slit-like opening in a patient's intramural course of the left coronary artery (LCA). Notice the normal round opening of the right coronary artery (RCA). The intraoperative image shows a probe within the intramural segment of the LCA

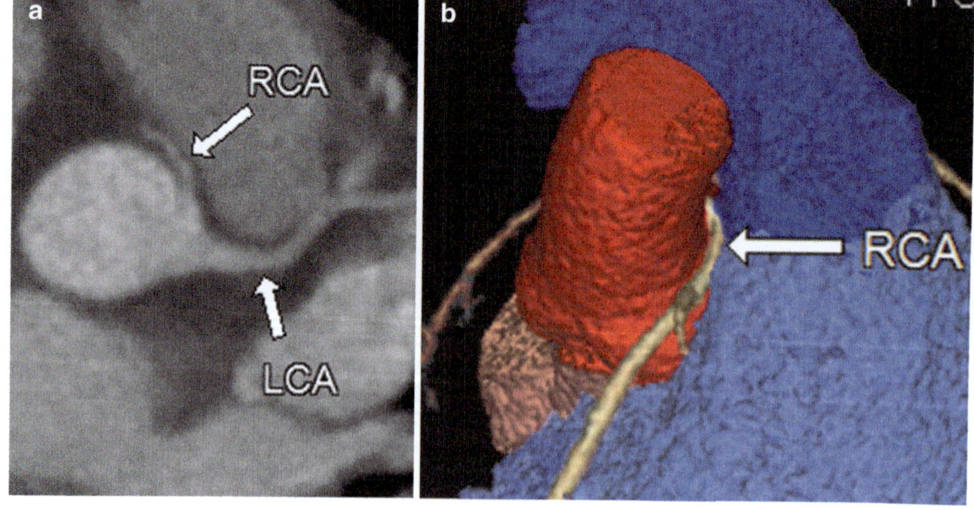

Fig. 5.14 Axial MIP image (**a**) and lateral 3D image (**b**) from a cardiac CTA in a child showing the right coronary artery (RCA) arising from the left coronary sinus and then coursing from left to right between the main pulmonary artery (*blue*) and the aorta (*red*). There is narrowing of the proximal RCA, and the patient showed an 8-mm intramural course along the wall of the aorta before exiting into the right atrioventricular groove

Fig. 5.15 Axial MIP image (**a**) and virtual angioscopy image (**b**) from a cardiac CTA of a child show the slit-like opening in a patient's intramural course of the right coronary artery (RCA). Notice the normal round opening of the left coronary artery (LCA)

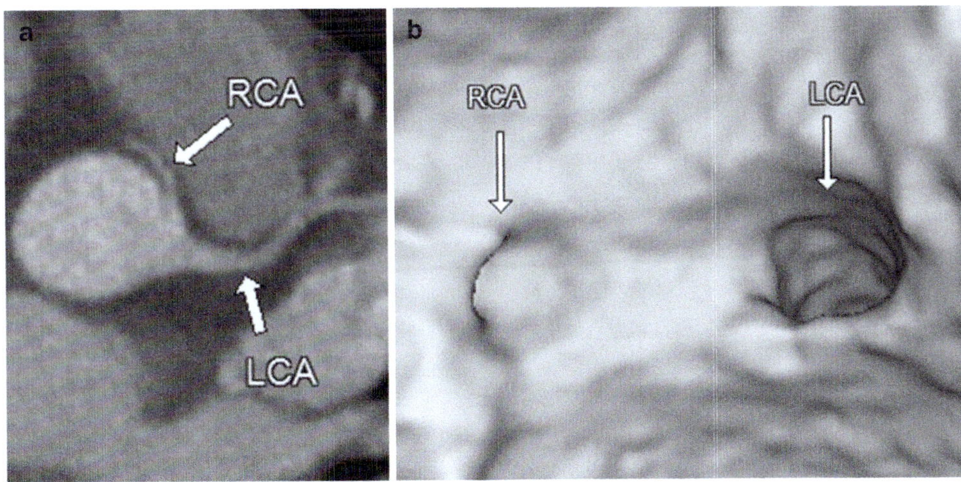

Fig. 5.16 A coronal image (**a**) and a virtual angioscopy image (**b**) from a cardiac CTA in a child show side-to-side narrowing of the proximal right coronal artery (RCA), and the patient showed an 8-mm intramural course along the wall of the aorta before exiting into a normal course. The increased height-width ratio of greater than 2:1 correlates well with an intramural course

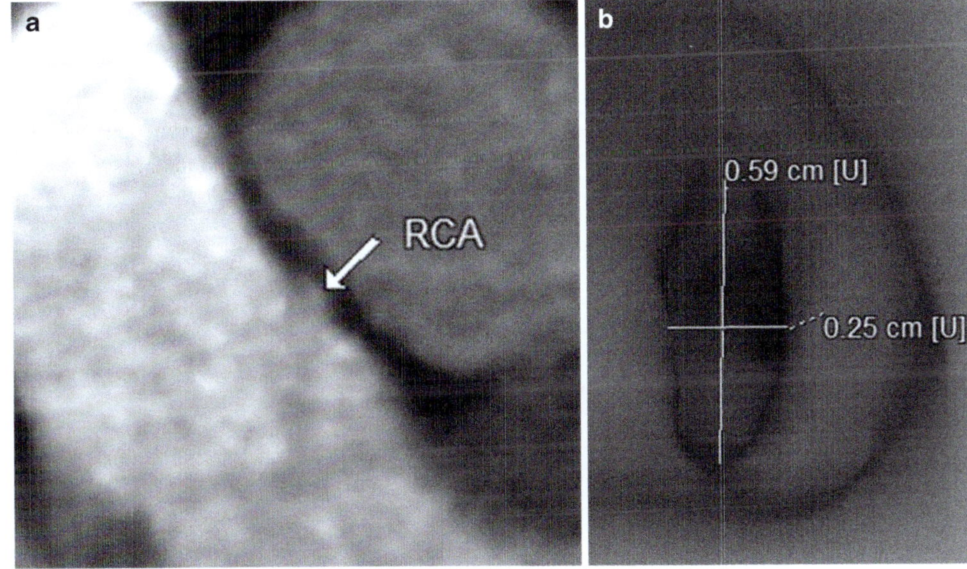

5.4   Trans-septal Course

The trans-septal course of the coronary artery is a well-described anomalous course typically seen when the left coronary artery arises from the right coronary sinus and then courses along the posterior right ventricular wall of the interventricular septum. The course is typically benign, although some case reports of compression have been described.

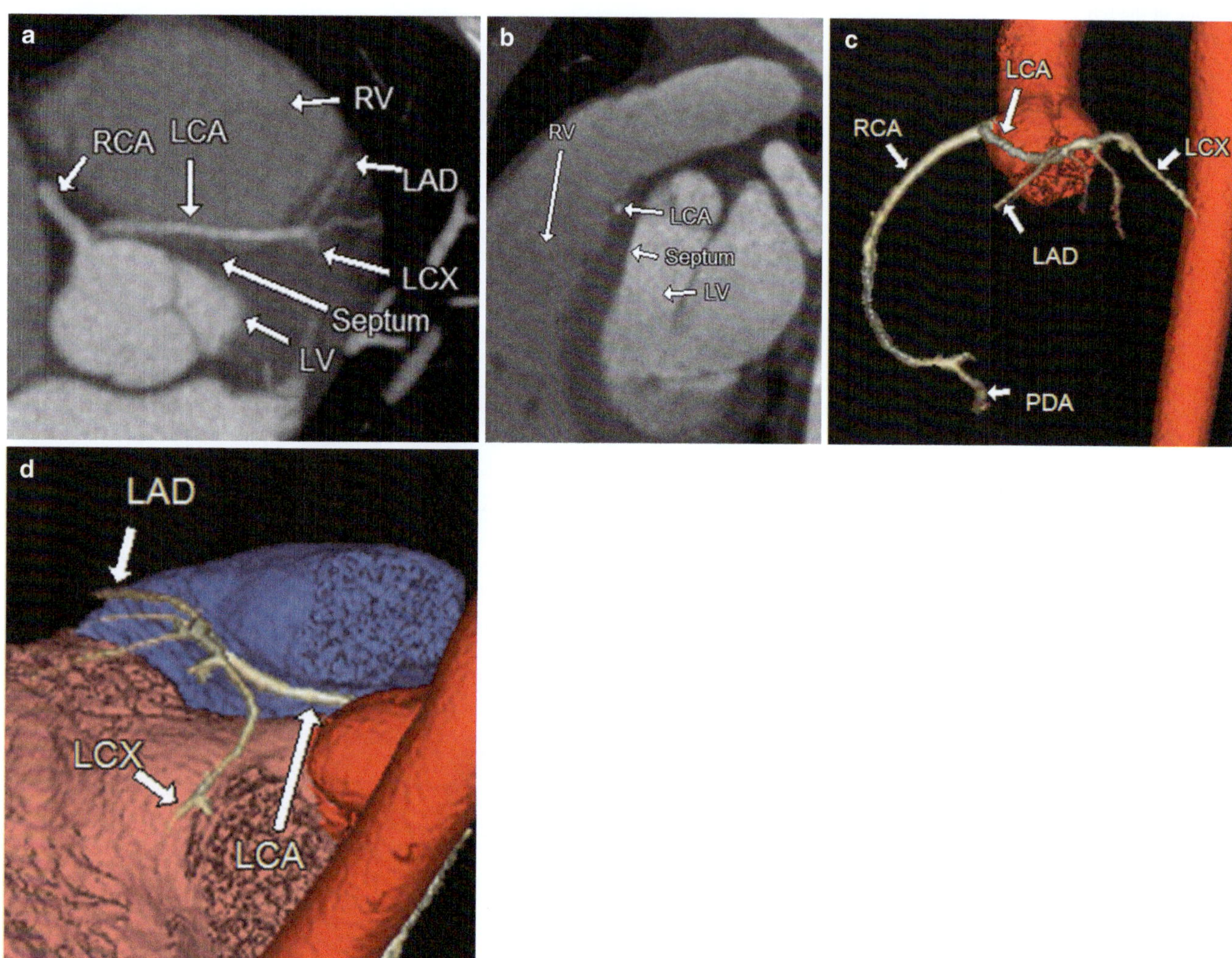

Fig. 5.17 Axial and sagittal MIP images (**a**, **b**) and 3D images (**c**, **d**) from a cardiac CTA in a child show the left coronary artery (LCA) arising from the right coronary sinus. It then courses along the posterior wall of the right ventricle (RV) within the interventricular septum between the right (RV) and left (LV) ventricles. Notice that the proximal LCA drops inferiorly. This is called the "hammock sign" and is consistent with a trans-septal course of the LCA

5.5   Myocardial Bridge

Normally, the coronaries are surrounded by epicardial fat and can course through the myocardium, which is called a myocardial bridge. Most patients with myocardial bridging are asymptomatic. The left anterior descending artery or LAD is the most common vessel to bridge the myocardium, although any coronary vessel can have an intramyocardial course. The depth of the bridging has shown differences in clinical significance.

5.6   Retro-cardiac

Another possible anomalous course of the coronary arteries crossing from right to left or left to right is a retro-cardiac course. In this anomaly, the coronary artery courses along the posterior atrioventricular (AV) groove behind the AV valves.

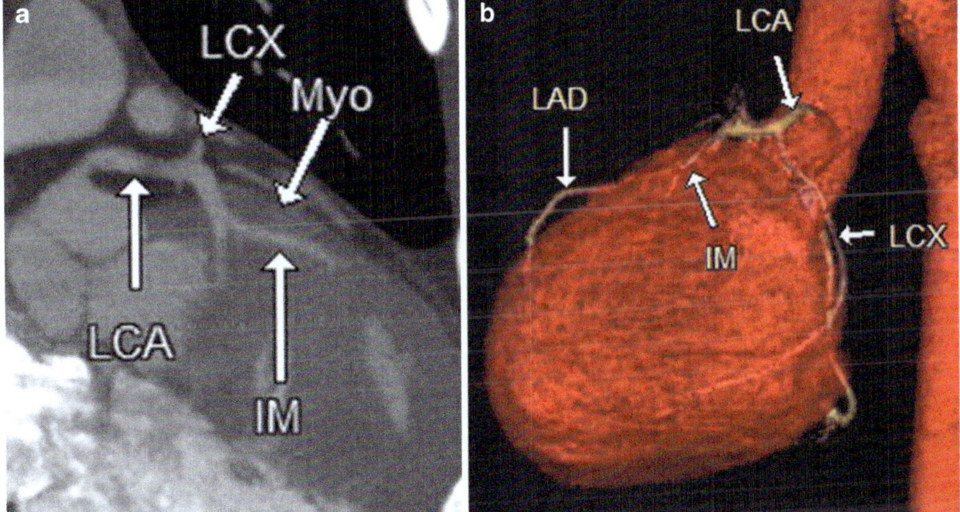

Fig. 5.18 Coronal MIP image (**a**) and 3D images (**b**) from a cardiac CTA in an child show a long segment of myocardial bridging of the LAD. The intramyocardial segment (IM) does narrow before exiting into the epicardial fat. The main left coronary (LCA) artery and circumflex artery (LCX) are labeled

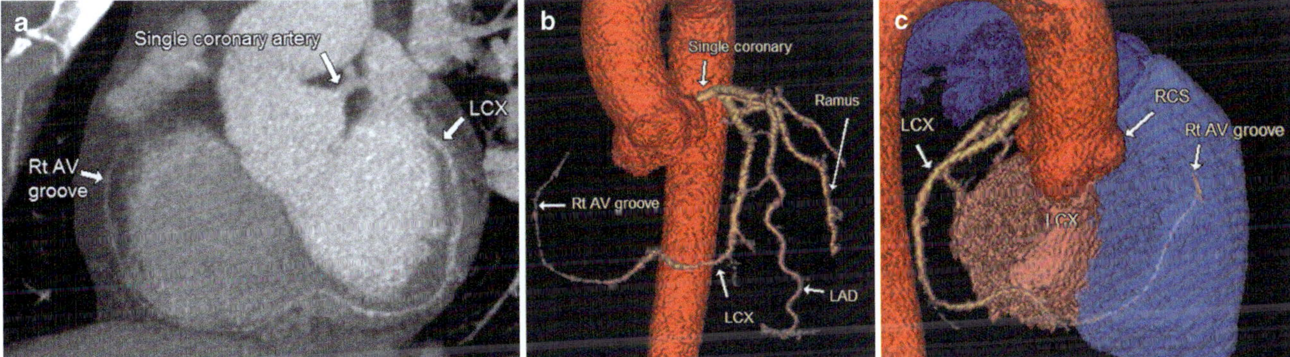

Fig. 5.19 Coronal MIP image (**a**) and 3D images (**b, c**) below from a cardiac CTA in a child show the absence of a right coronary artery. A single coronary artery arises from the left coronary sinus with an elon-gated course of the circumflex artery (LCX) along the posterior atrio-ventricular (AV) grove until it reaches the right AV grove in the normal position of a right coronary artery

Suggested Reading

Angelini P, Walmsley RP, Libreros A, Ott DA. Symptomatic anomalous origination of the left coronary artery from the opposite sinus of valsalva. Clinical presentations, diagnosis, and surgical repair. Tex Heart Inst J. 2006;33:171–9.

Cacici G, Angelini P. Unusual case of single coronary artery: questions of methods and basic concepts. Ital Heart J. 2005;6:345–7.

Dodge-Khatami A, Mavroudis C, Backer CL. Congenital Heart Surgery Nomenclature and Database Project: anomalies of the coronary arteries. Ann Thorac Surg. 2000;69:S270–S97.

Ferreira AG Jr, Trotter SE, König B Jr, Décourt LV, Fox K, Olsen EG. Myocardial bridges: morphological and functional aspects. Br Heart J. 1991;66:364–7.

Miller JA, Anavekar NS, El Yaman MM, Burkhart HM, Miller AJ, Julsrud PR. Computed tomographic angiography identification of intramural segments in anomalous coronary arteries with interarterial course. Int J Cardiovasc Imaging. 2012;28:1525–32.

Villa AD, Sammut E, Nair A, Rajani R, Bonamini R, Chiribiri A. Coronary artery anomalies overview: the normal and the abnormal. World J Radiol. 2016;28(8):537–55.

Evaluating the course of coronary arteries in patients with congenital heart disease can have important implications for future surgical interventions. We review examples of patients with congenital heart disease with coronary anomalies that have clinically significant impact (Figs. 6.1, 6.2, 6.3, 6.4, 6.5, and 6.6).

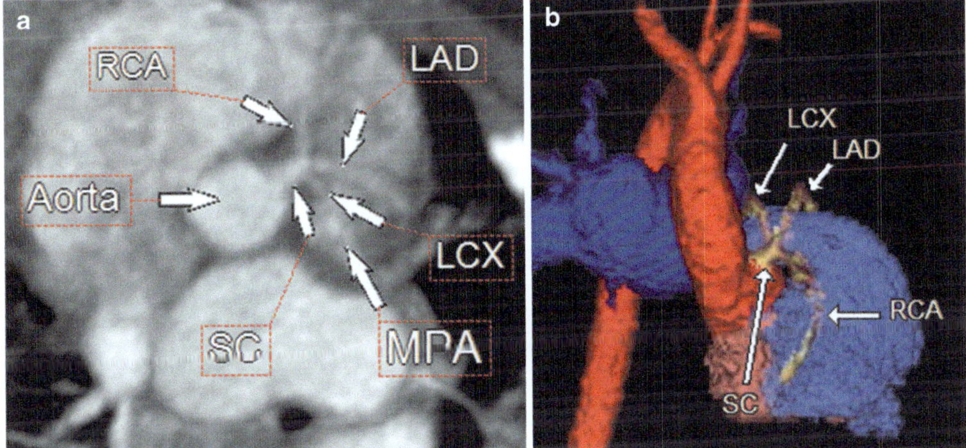

Fig. 6.1 Axial maximum intensity project (MIP) (**a**) and 3D volume-rendered image (**b**) from a cardiac computed tomography angiograph (CTA) in an infant with Tetralogy of Fallot and absent pulmonic valve demonstrates a single coronary (SC) artery arising from the right coronary sinus. Notice the significant clockwise rotation of the aortic root which positions the right coronary sinus to the left of midline. The left anterior descending (LAD) and left circumflex (LCX) course anterior and superrior to the pulmonary outlfow tract (purple). This course is important to identify as the surgeon will need to take this into account when creating an right ventrical (RV) to pulmonary artery (PA) conduit. Obviously, severing the LAD and LCX is a potential risk in this patient if the surgeon is not advised

© Springer Nature Switzerland AG 2020
R. R. Richardson, *Atlas of Pediatric CTA of Coronary Artery Anomalies*, https://doi.org/10.1007/978-3-030-28087-1_6

Fig. 6.2 Postoperative axial MIP (**a**) and 3D volume-rendered image (**b**) from a cardiac CTA in an infant with Tetralogy of Fallot and absent pulmonic valve showing the RV to PA conduit (RV-PA) created anterior to the anomalous course of the LAD and LCX from the single coronary artery (SC)

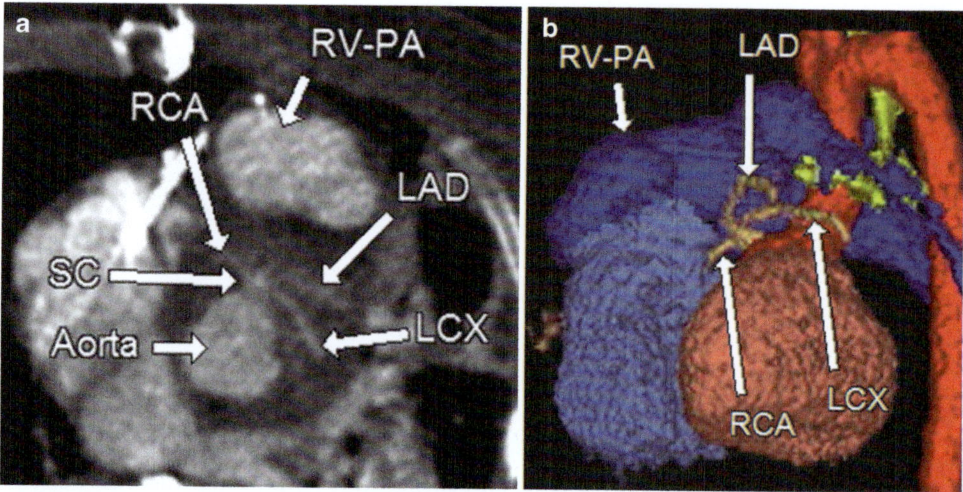

Fig. 6.3 Axial MIP (**a**) and 3D volume-rendered image (**b**) from a cardiac CTA in an infant with double outlet right ventricle. The right (RCA) and left (LCA) coronary arteries arise from the right coronary sinus. The left coronary (LCA) courses anterior to the main pulmonary artery (MPA) before branching into LAD and LCX. Notice that the right ventricle (purple) supplies both the aorta (red) and the main pulmonary artery (MPA, blue) consistent with double outlet right ventricle

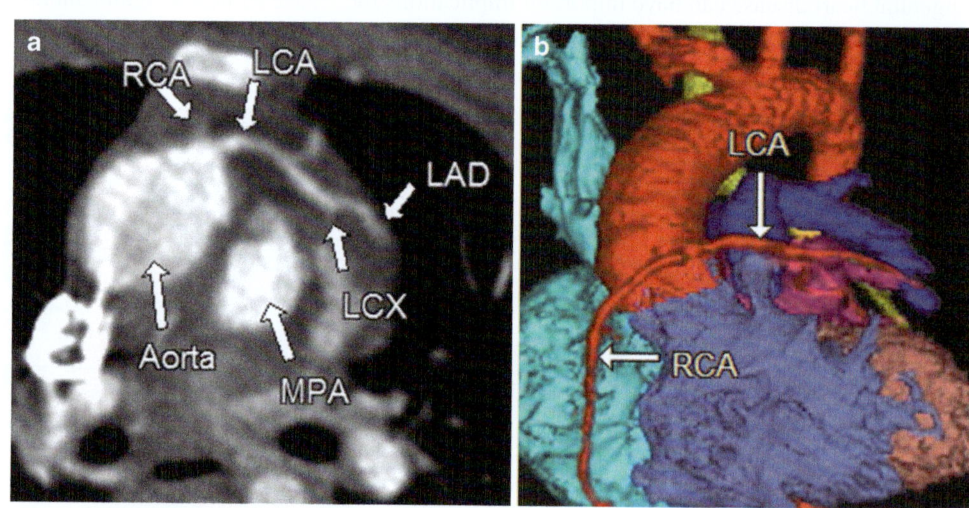

Fig. 6.4 Postoperative axial MIP (**a**) and 3D volume-rendered image (**b**) from a cardiac CTA in an infant with double outlet right ventricle shows RV to PA conduit anterior to the anomlaous course of the left coronary artery arising from the right coronary sinus. The LAD and LCX are shown. The right coronary artery (RCA) has a normal course

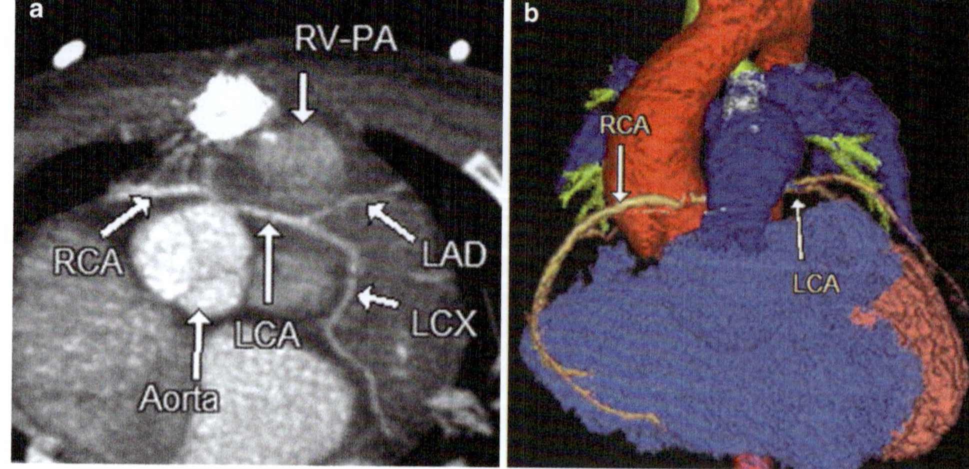

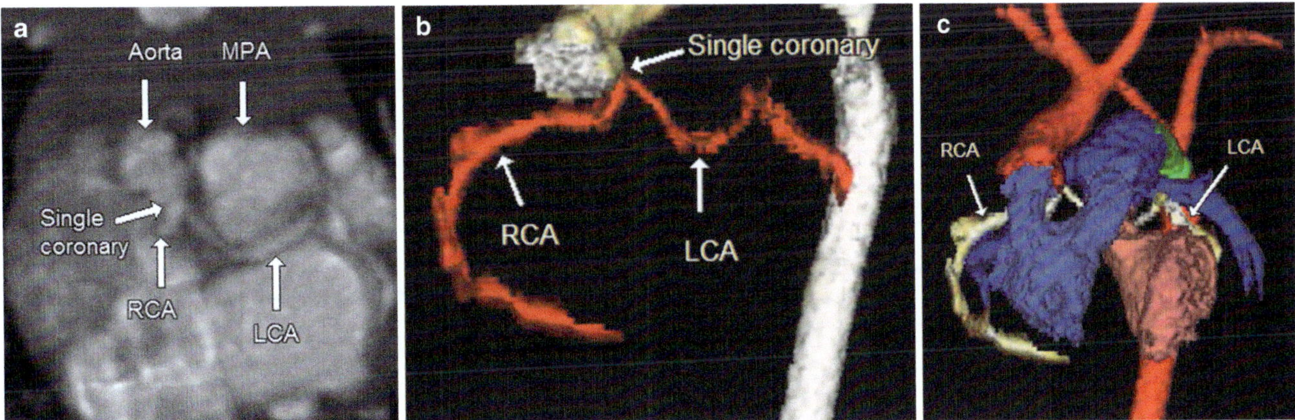

Fig. 6.5 Axial MIP (**a**) and 3D volume-rendered image (**b**) from a cardiac CTA in an infant with double outlet right ventricle and a single coronary artery from the left coronary sinus. (**c**) Notice the elongated course of the left coronary artery (LCA) that courses posterior and infc-rior to the main pulmonary artery (MPA) while the right coronary artery (RCA) courses posterior to and around the aorta. This is favorable anatomy as the coronaries will not be in the way of needed repairs

Fig. 6.6 Postoperative axial MIP (**a**) and 3D volume-rendered image (**b**) from a cardiac CTA in an infant with a history of transposition of the great vessels status after arterial switch (notice how the right and left pulmonary arteries straddle the ascending aorta). After tranloscation of the coronaries the left coronary artery (LCA) was compressed by the aorta and main pulmonary artery (MPA) causing clinically significant stenosis

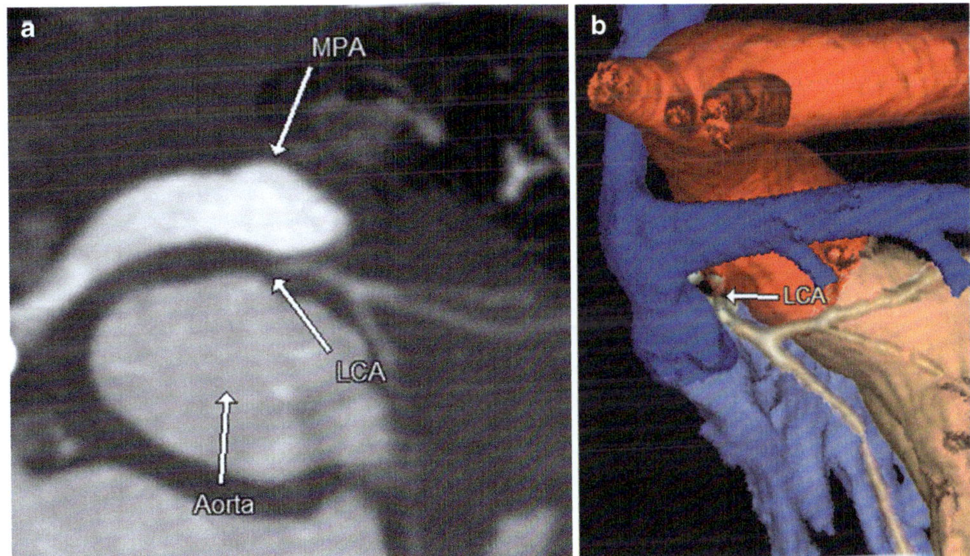

Suggested Reading

Enaba MM, Hasan DI, Alsowey AM, Elsayed H. Multidetector computed tomography(CT) in evaluation of congenital cyanotic heart diseases. Pol J Radiol. 2017;82:645–59.

Gulati GS, Singh C, Kothari SS, Sharma S. An unusual coronary artery anomaly in tetralogy of Fallot shown on MDCT. AJR Am J Roentgenol. 2006;186(4):1192–3.

Kochar A, Kiefer T. Coronary artery anomalies: when you need to worry. Curr Cardiol Rep 2017;19(5):39. https://doi.org/10.1007/s11886-017-0854-x. Review

Coronary artery fistulas are anomalies of termination of the coronary arteries. Coronary artery fistulas are defined by a direct precapillary connection between a branch of a coronary artery and the lumen of a chamber of the heart or great vessel, typically pulmonary artery or inferior vena cava (IVC). These fistulas more commonly terminate in a lower pressure chamber of the heart such as the right ventricle or right atrium or a low-pressure great vessel such as the pulmonary artery or IVC. The coronary fistula to the right ventricle is most common (41%) [1] with termination into the right atrium accounting for 26% and pulmonary artery 17% [1].

Branches of the right coronary artery are slightly more likely to form coronary fistulas (50%), with both branches of the left coronary artery representing 42% of the time both coronary arteries had fistulous branches [1].

Patients are typically asymptomatic with symptoms most likely due to left to right shunting. Fistulas are most frequently detected with a continuous murmur and the fistula is found on a subsequent echocardiogram. Computed tomography angiography (CTA) or angiography is typically used to delineate the fistula.

Patients with pulmonic atresia with an intact ventricular septum more frequently develop fistulas due to the increased pressure in the right ventricle. These coronary artery fistulas are often referred to as sinusoids. The myocardium may be supplied by these sinusoids resulting in deoxygenated blood supplying the muscle tissue. Myocardial infarction may develop. The other risk when sinusoids are present is for a myocardial steal with flow coursing toward the lower pressure right ventricle. Physiologic flow depends on the pressure of the right ventricle (Figs. 7.1, 7.2, 7.3, 7.4, 7.5, 7.6, 7.7, and 7.8).

© Springer Nature Switzerland AG 2020
R. R. Richardson, *Atlas of Pediatric CTA of Coronary Artery Anomalies*, https://doi.org/10.1007/978-3-030-28087-1_7

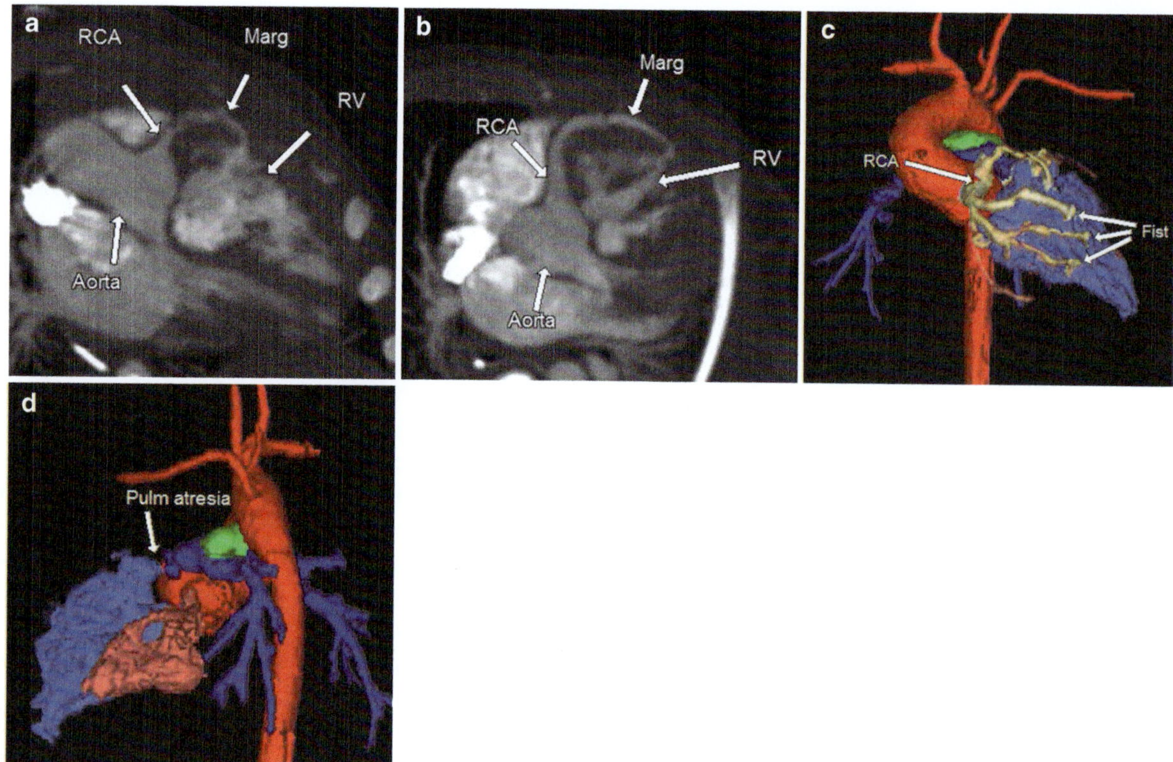

Fig. 7.1 Two axial maximum intensity projection (MIP) images (**a**, **b**) and two 3D volume-rendered images (**c**, **d**) from a cardiac CTA in an infant with pulmonic atresia and an intact ventricular septum. Images show multiple marginal branches (Marg) of the right coronary artery (RCA) communicating directly with the right ventricle consistent with coronary fistulas (Fist) or sinusoids. This is commonly seen in patients with pulmonic atresia and an intact ventricular septum as the right ventricle is "pressurized"

Fig. 7.2 Single 3D volume-rendered image from a cardiac CTA in an infant with pulmonic atresia and an intact ventricular septum. Images show multiple fistulas (Fist) from both the right (RCA) and left (LCA) coronary arteries communicating with the right ventricle consistent with coronary fistulas (Fist) or sinusoids. This is common in patients with pulmonic atresia and an intact ventricular septum as the right ventricle is "pressurized"

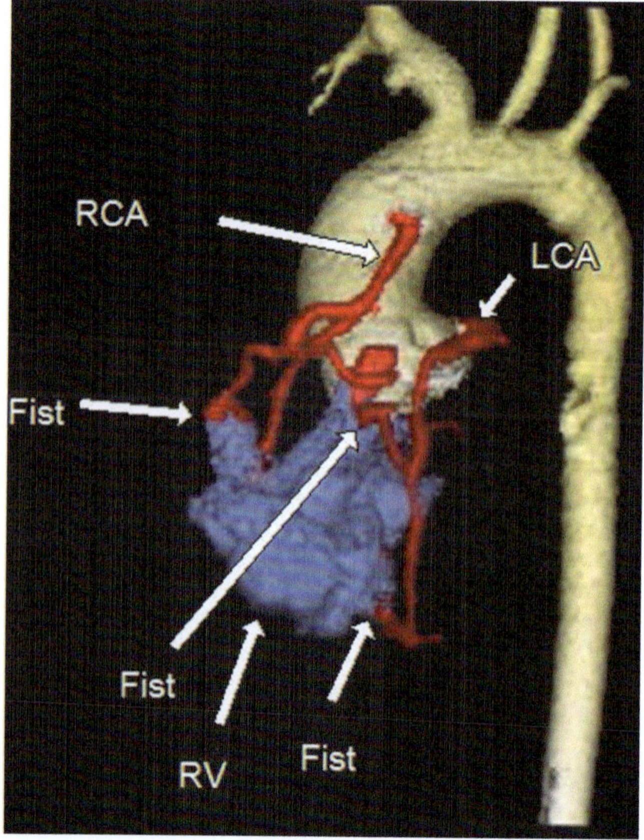

Fig. 7.3 Oblique axial MIP image (**a**) and a 3D volume-rendered image (**b**) from a cardiac CTA in a 6 month old patient who presented with a continuous murmur. Images show massive enlargement of the right coronary artery (RCA) with a blush of contrast into the right atrium (RA) consistent with a coronary artery fistula to the right atrium. Notice the normal or slightly diminuitive size of the left coronary artery (LCA)

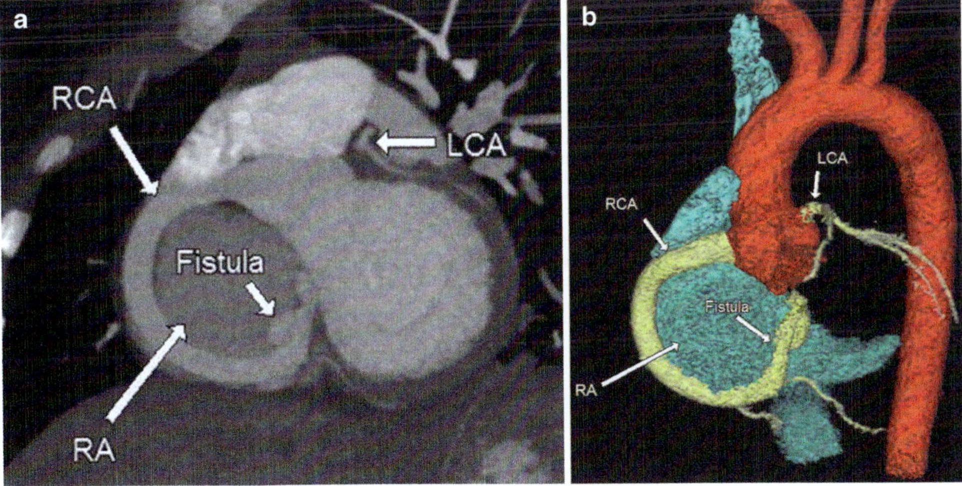

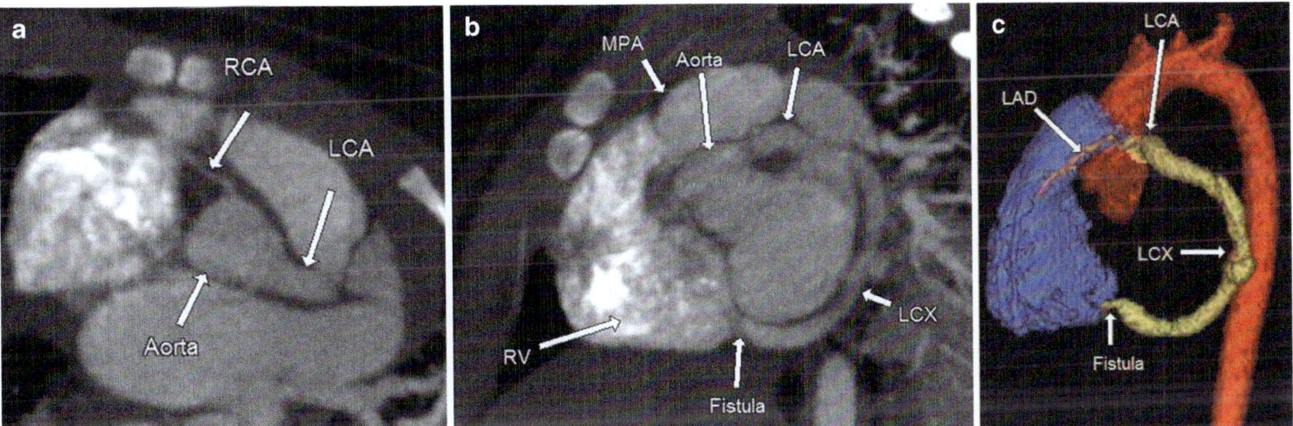

Fig. 7.4 Axial (**a**) and oblique (**b**) MIP images and a 3D volume-rendered image (**c**) from a cardiac CTA in a 3-day old patient who presented with a continuous murmur. Images show massive enlargement of the left coronary artery (LCA) with direct communication distally with the right ventricle (RV) consistent with a coronary artery fistula to the right ventricle. Notice the normal or slightly diminuitive size of the right coronary artery (RCA)

Fig. 7.5 Oblique MIP image (**a**) and a 3D volume-rendered image (**b**) from a cardiac CTA in a 16-year-old patient who presented with atypical chest pain. Images show multiple collaterals arising from the right coronary artery (RCA) that eventually communicate with the pulmonary artery (blue) consistent with a coronary artery fistula to the pulmonary artery. Notice the normal or slightly diminuitive size of the left coronary artery (LCA)

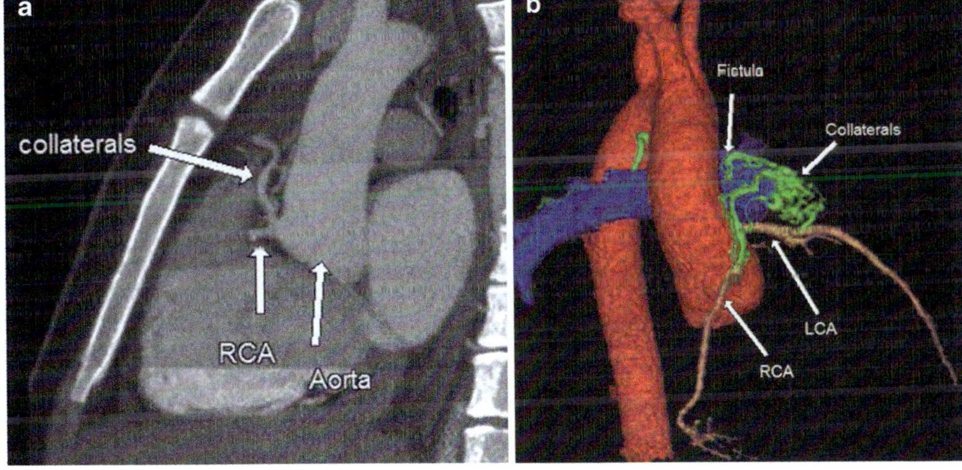

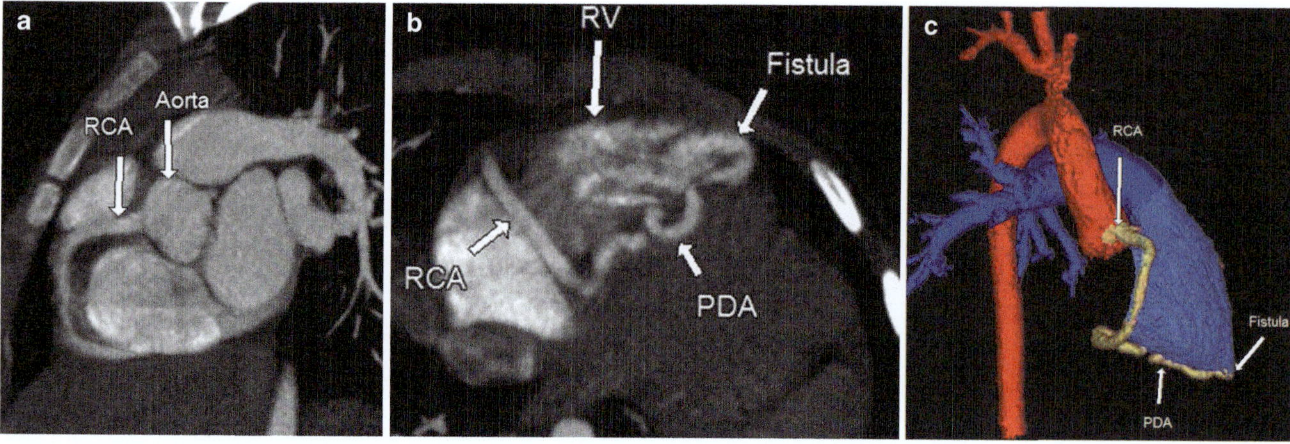

Fig. 7.6 Oblique (**A**) and axial (**B**) MIP images and a 3D volume-rendered image (**C**) from a cardiac CTA in a 3-year-old patient who presented to the pediatrician with a continuous murmur. Images show enlargement of the right coronary artery (RCA) with communication distally with the inferior left side of the right ventricle (RV) consistent with a coronary artery fistula to the right ventricle. Notice the tortuous prominent course of the right coronary and posterior descending artery (PDA)

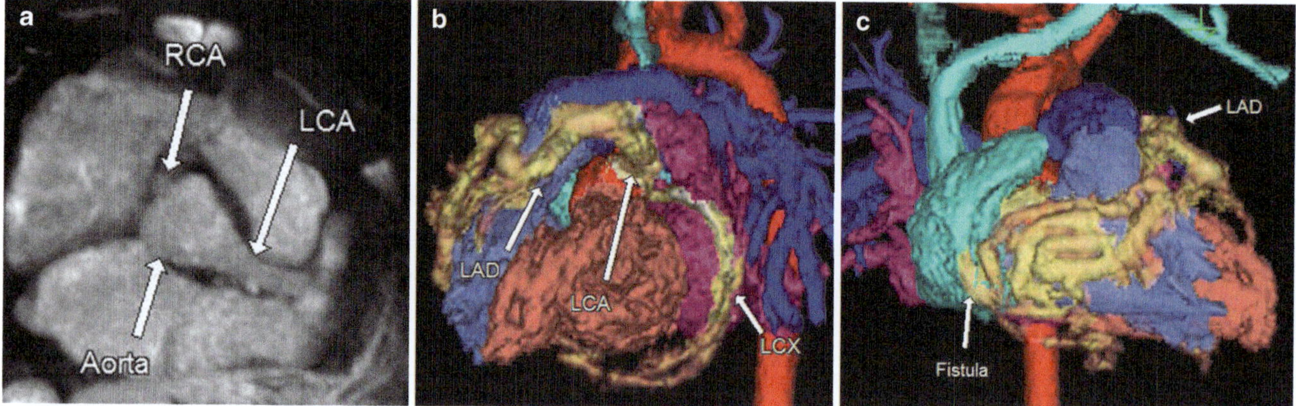

Fig. 7.7 Axial MIP image (**a**) and a 3D volume-rendered images (**b, c**) from a cardiac CTA in a 2-month-old patient who presented with a continuous murmur. Images show massive enlargement and tortuosity of the left anterior descending coronary artery (LAD) with a blush of contrast into the right atrium (light blue) consistent with a coronary artery fistula to the right atrium. Notice the normal size of the left circumflex coronary artery (LCX) and right coronary artery (RCA)

Fig. 7.8 Oblique axial MIP image (**a**) and a 3D volume-rendered image (**b**) from a cardiac CTA in an 8-year-old patient who presented with atypical chest pain. Images show prominence of a branch of the left coronary artery (LCA) which communicates with the main pulmonary artery (blue) consistent with a coronary artery fistula to the pulmonary artery. There was increased left to right shunt

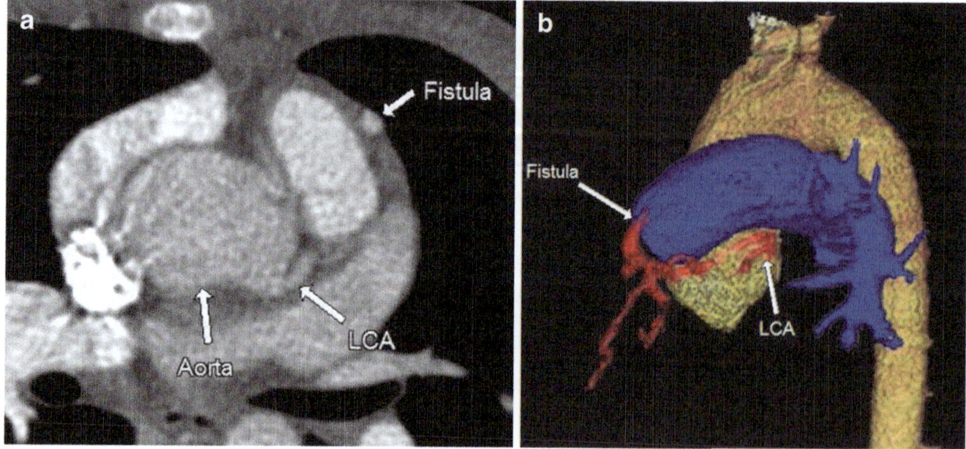

References

1. Andropoulos DB, Gottlieb EA. Pulmonary atresia with intact ventricular septum. In: Gatzoulis M, Webb G, Daubeney P, editors. Diagnosis and management of adult congenital heart disease. 2nd ed. London: Churchill Livingstone; 2012. p. 339–46.

Suggested Reading

Gowda RM, Vasavada BC, Khan IA. Coronary artery fistulas: clinical and therapeutic considerations. Int J Cardiol. 2006;107(1):7–10.

Mavroudis C, Backer CL, Rocchini AP, Muster AJ, Gevitz M. Coronary artery fistulas in infants and children: a surgical review and discussion of coil embolization. Ann Thorac Surg. 1997;63(5):1235–42.

Schmitt R, Froehner S, Brunn J, Wagner M, Brunner H, Cherevatyy O, et al. Congenital anomalies of the coronary arteries: imaging with contrast-enhanced, multi-detector computed tomography. Eur Radiol. 2005;15(6):1110–21. Epub 2005 Mar 9

Schumacher G, Roithmaier A, Lorenz HP, Meisner H, Sauer U, Müller KD, et al. Congenital coronary artery fistula in infancy and childhood: diagnostic and therapeutic aspects. Thorac Cardiovasc Surg. 1997;45(6):287–94.

Shirani J, Brofferio A. Isolated coronary artery anomalies. http://www.emedicine.com/med/topic445.htm. March 13, 2008.

Coronary Artery Abnormalities in Patients with Kawasaki Disease and Williams Syndrome

8.1 Kawasaki Disease

The most common and serious complications of Kawasaki disease are coronary artery abnormalities. In patients with Kawasaki disease, coronary artery involvement is seen in approximately 15–20% of patients [1]. Over the years, the definition of coronary artery involvement has varied but it is now defined by internal lumen diameter, adjusted to body surface area Z-scores Table 8.1 [2–4].

Coronary artery abnormalities typically reside within left anterior descending and proximal right coronary arteries. However, abnormalities are also seen in the left main coronary artery, circumflex, and distal right coronary artery [3]. Figure 8.1 illustrates a patient who has multiple right coronary aneurysms. In patients who have coronary artery involvement, the proximal vessels are almost always involved before distal segments. The shapes and sizes of the coronary artery abnormalities can change and evolve over time. How the abnormality evolves largely depends on how aggressive the disease presented during the acute phase of illness. Aneurysms can increase in size up to 6 weeks after disease onset and can regress within 2 years.

Around 50–75% of aneurysms decrease to a normal lumen diameter, especially those that are minimally dilated or inflamed [5]. However, large or giant coronary artery aneurysms do not resolve because they have lost the intima blood vessel layer [1, 2]. These include the aneurysms that are ≥8 mm in diameter or have a Z-score ≥10. Most of these aneurysms contain thrombi and are prone to cause myocardial infarctions. Furthermore, with time, these thrombi can calcify, making rupture less likely. Figure 8.2 nicely depicts calcified and non calcified coronary aneurysms. Importantly, patients who have large or giant coronary artery aneurysms can also develop aneurysms in the axillary, brachial, and subclavian arteries, especially near their branch points; however, thromboses at these sites are rare [6].

Notably, most patients with coronary artery involvement lie within the dilation-only category, whose Z-scores are normal but have luminal diameters that are out of the

Table 8.1 Depicts the current classification system for coronary artery abnormalities seen in patients with Kawasaki disease [2–4]

Classification	Z-Score
No coronary involvement	Z-score always <2 **and** no more than a 0.9 decrease in Z-score during follow-up
Dilation only	Z-score 2 to <2.5 **or** if initially <2, a ≥ 1 decrease in Z-score during follow-up; these patients have luminal measurements outside of normal range
Small aneurysm	Z-score ≥2.5 to <5
Medium aneurysm	Z-score of ≥5 to <10 **and** absolute dimension <8 mm
Large or giant aneurysm	Z-score ≥10 **or** absolute dimension ≥8 mm

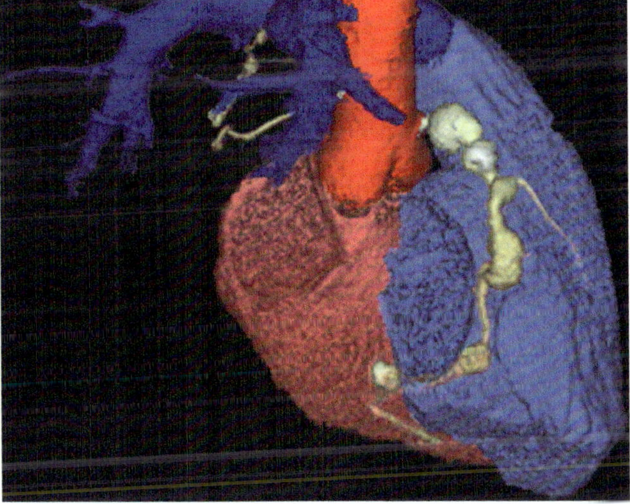

Fig. 8.1 Multiple right coronary artery aneurysms (tan) are shown along the right atrioventricular groove in a child with Kawasaki's disease. The aorta (red), pulmonary arteries (blue), left ventricle (salmon), and right ventricle (purple) are also shown

normal range. These patients may present with normal coronary artery dimensions, but with follow up, are subsequently found to have decreasing dimensions over time. This suggests that their coronary artery was dilated initially. Patients in the dilation-only category commonly

© Springer Nature Switzerland AG 2020
R. R. Richardson, *Atlas of Pediatric CTA of Coronary Artery Anomalies*, https://doi.org/10.1007/978-3-030-28087-1_8

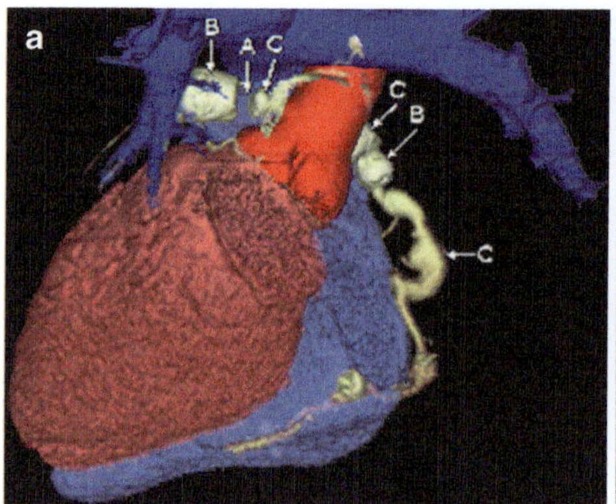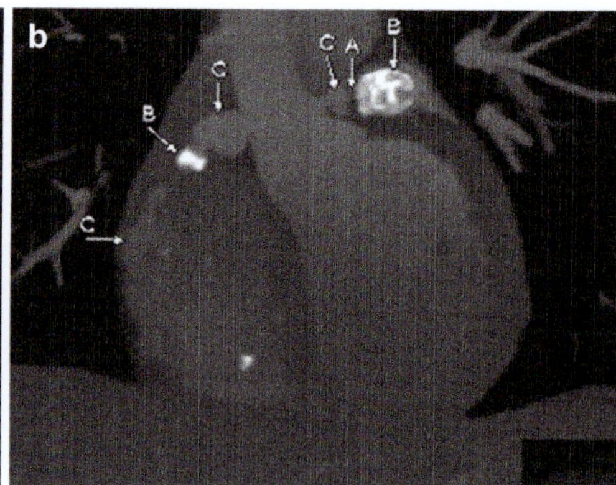

Fig. 8.2 Maximum intensity projection (MIP) image (**a**) and posterior view from a 3D color-coded computed tomography angiogram (CTA) (**b**) in a 13-year-old patient with history of Kawasaki disease shows calcified (B) and non-calcified (C) coronary aneurysms. Note complete occlusion of the left coronary artery (A)

resolve their dilation within 4–8 weeks [2]. Overall, coronary artery aneurysms resolve more commonly the younger the child is at more distal sites [7]. Fusiform coronary aneurysms more commonly resolve as well.

Some patients are at higher risk for having an associated coronary artery abnormality. These include a late diagnosis and delayed treatment with intravenous immunoglobulin (IVIG), age <1 year and age >9 years, male individuals, individuals of Asian, Pacific Islander, and Hispanic race, long duration of fever, and failure to respond to initial IVIG treatment [8].

8.2 Coronary Artery Involvement in Patients with Williams Syndrome

Williams Syndrome (WS), a heterozygous deletion on chromosome 7q11.23, involves a deletion of the elastin gene and frequently manifests with cardiovascular abnormalities secondary to elastin haploinsufficiency [9]. Supravalvular aortic stenosis (SVAS), pulmonic valve stenosis, and coronary artery abnormalities are most common [10].

In the arterial system, elastin accounts for the reversible distensibility of arteries and allows for vascular recoil [10]. The hemizygosity of the elastin gene in patients with WS leads to increased stiffness in arterial vessels [11]. Elastin also modulates the migration of smooth muscle cells. In the absence of elastin, subendothelial migration and proliferation of smooth muscle occurs to a degree that results in widespread stenosis of the vascular lumen [10].

SVAS is the most common cardiovascular lesion in WS, presenting in up to 75% of cases [10]. SVAS may develop either as a discrete, hourglass narrowing at the sinotubular junction, or a long-segment diffuse stenosis of the ascending aorta (Fig. 8.3) [10]. Although SVAS may occur in isolation, it is often associated with pulmonary artery stenosis, coronary ostial stenosis or dilation, stenosis of the brachiocephalic vessels, and aortic valve abnormalities [10].

Recent studies estimate the incidence of pulmonary artery stenosis in WS at 40%, and diffuse stenosis is typically seen at the branches of peripheral pulmonary arteries [10]. Supravalvular pulmonary stenosis may occur, but significantly less frequently; occurring only in 12% of all patients with WS [12]. Patients with pulmonary artery stenosis in WS typically see an improvement in pulmonary blood flow over time, as pulmonary artery elastin physiologically decreases in the first few months of life while pulmonary vascular resistance is normalizing [10].

Of the patients with WS that have SVAS, 45% of them also have coronary artery involvement. Such coronary artery involvement may present as diffuse coronary artery stenosis, coronary artery dilation, obstruction to coronary artery inflow by the aortic valve, or coronary ostial stenosis [13]. Supravalvular aortic narrowing generates hemodynamic turbulence in the aortic root just beneath the sinotubular junction, and likely contributes to the development of coronary ostial stenosis. Such coronary ostial stenosis is the most commonly reported coronary abnormality in WS in recent literature, occurring in up to 9% of patients within the first year of life [13]. Adhesions of the abnormal aortic leaflet edges to the narrowed sinotubular junction may also impair inflow to the coronary arteries [13]. In this setting, the coronary ostia undergo intimal proliferation, accounting for critical narrowing of the coronary origin [14]. Alternatively, high pressure proximal to the SVAS in some instances may be transmitted to the coronary arteries, resulting in severe dysplasia and narrowing [10].

Fig. 8.3 Oblique coronal MIP image (**a**) and 3D volume-rendered image (**b**) in a child with known WS. There is diffuse coronary stenosis of the right coronary artery (RCA) and marked dilatation of the left coronary artery (LCA). Notice the severe supravalvular aortic stenosis (SVAS) classically seen in patients with WS

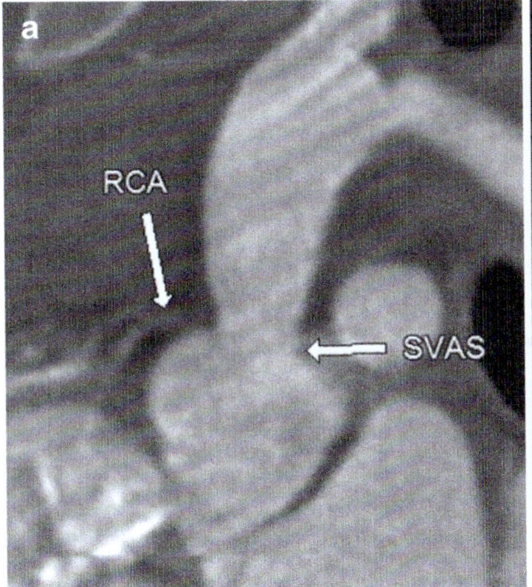

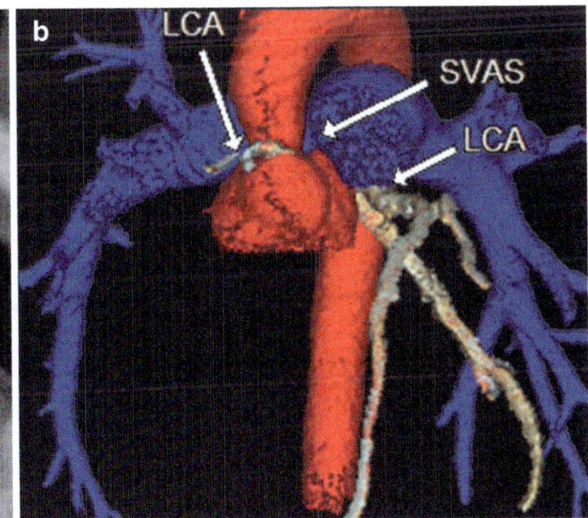

References

1. Ghelani S, Kwatra N, Spurney C. Can coronary artery involvement in Kawasaki disease be predicted? Diagnostics. 2013;3(2):232–43.
2. McCrindle BW, Rowley AH, Newburger JW, Burns JC, Bolger AF, Gewitz M, et al. Diagnosis, treatment, and long-term management of Kawasaki disease: a scientific statement for health professionals from the American Heart Association. Circulation. 2017;135:e927–99. Epub 2017 Mar 29
3. Kitamura S, Kameda Y, Seki T, Kawachi K, Endo M, Takeuchi Y, et al. Long-term outcome of myocardial revascularization in patients with Kawasaki coronary artery disease. A multicenter cooperative study. J Thorac Cardiovasc Surg. 1994;107:663–73; discussion 673–4
4. Manlhiot C, Millar K, Golding F, McCrindle BW. Improved classification of coronary artery abnormalities based only on coronary artery z-scores after Kawasaki disease. Pediatr Cardiol. 2010;31:242–9.
5. Kato H, Sugimura T, Akagi T, Sato N, Hashino K, Maeno Y, et al. Long-term consequences of Kawasaki disease. A 10- to 21-year follow-up study of 594 patients. Circulation. 1996;94:1379–85.
6. Orenstein JM, Shulman ST, Fox LM, Baker SC, Takahashi M, Bhatti TR, et al. Three linked vasculo-pathic processes characterize Kawasaki disease: a light and trans- mission electron microscopic study. PLoS One. 2012;7:e38998. https://doi.org/10.1371/journal.pone.0038998.
7. Takahashi M, Mason W, Lewis AB. Regression of coronary aneurysms in patients with Kawasaki syndrome. Circulation. 1987;75:387–94.
8. Belay ED, Maddox RA, Holman RC, Curns AT, Ballah K, Schonberger LB. Kawasaki syndrome and risk factors for coronary artery abnormalities: United States, 1994–2003. Pediatr Infect Dis J. 2006;25:245–9.
9. Morris CA. Introduction: Williams syndrome. Am J Med Genet C Semin Med Genet. 2010;154C(2):203–8. https://doi.org/10.1002/ajmg.c.30266.
10. Thomas Collins R. Cardiovascular disease in Williams syndrome. Curr Opin Pediatr. 2018;30(5):609–15.
11. Salaymeh KJ, Banerjee A. Evaluation of arterial stiffness in children with Williams syndrome: does it play a role in evolving hypertension? Am Heart J. 2001;142:549–55.
12. Collins RT 2nd, Kaplan P, Somes GW, Rome JJ. Cardiovascular abnormalities, interventions, and long-term outcomes in infantile Williams syndrome. J Pediatr. 2010;156:253–8.e1.
13. Federici D, Ranghetti A, Merlo M, Terzi A, Di Dedda GB, Marcora S, et al. Coronary artery involvement of williams syndrome in infants and surgical revascularization strategy. Ann Thorac Surg. 2016;101(1):359–61.
14. Stamm C, Friehs I, Ho SY, Moran AM, Jonas RA, del Nido PJ. Congenital supravalvular aortic stenosis: a simple lesion? Eur J Cardiothorac Surg. 2001;19:195–202.

Index

© Springer Nature Switzerland AG 2020

R. R. Richardson, *Atlas of Pediatric CTA of Coronary Artery Anomalies*, https://doi.org/10.1007/978-3-030-28087-1